Handbook of Early Pregnancy Care

Edited by

TOM BOURNE PhD FRCOG
Early Pregnancy, Gynaecological Ultrasound and MAS Unit
St George's, University of London
London
UK

GEORGE CONDOUS MRCOG FRANZCOG
Early Pregnancy Unit, Nepean Hospital
Western Clinical School, Nepean Campus
University of Sydney
Sydney
Australia

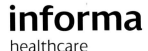
informa
healthcare

First published in the United Kingdom in 2006 by Informa Healthcare Ltd, 4 Park Square, Milton Park, Abingdon, Oxon OX14 4RN
Informa Healthcare is a trading division of Informa UK Ltd
Registered Office: 37/41 Mortimer Street, London W1T 3JH.
Registered in England and Wales Number 1072954.

Tel: +44 (0)20 7017 6000
Fax: +44 (0)20 7017 6699
Email: info.medicine@tandf.co.uk
Website: www.informahealthcare.com

Second printing 2007

A CIP record for this book is available from the British Library.
Library of Congress Cataloging-in-Publication Data

Data available on application

ISBN-10: 1 84214 323 9
ISBN-13: 978 1 84214 323 0

Distributed in North and South America by
Taylor & Francis
6000 Broken Sound Parkway, NW, (Suite 300)
Boca Raton, FL 33487, USA

Within Continental USA
Tel: 1 (800) 272 7737; Fax: 1 (800) 374 3401
Outside Continental USA
Tel: (561) 994 0555; Fax: (561) 361 6018
Email: orders@crcpress.com

Distributed in the rest of the world by
Thomson Publishing Services
Cheriton House
North Way
Andover, Hampshire SP10 5BE, UK
Tel: +44 (0)1264 332424
Email: tps.tandfsalesorder@thomson.com

Composition by Scribe Design Ltd, Ashford, Kent, UK
Printed and bound in India by Replika Press Pvt Ltd

Contents

Contributors

Maha Alkatib MRCOG
Early Pregnancy, Gynaecological Ultrasound
    and MAS Unit
St George's, University of London
London
UK

Cecilia Bottomley MRCOG
Early Pregnancy, Gynaecological Ultrasound
    and MAS Unit
St George's, University of London
London
UK

George Condous MRCOG FRANZCOG
Early Pregnancy Unit, Nepean Hospital
Western Clinical School, Nepean Campus
University of Sydney
Sydney
Australia

Steven R Goldstein MD
Professor of Obstetrics and Gynecology
New York University School of Medicine
New York, NY
USA

Seth Granberg MD PhD
Centre of Fetal Medicine and Gynecological
    Ultrasound
Department of Women's and Children's
    Health
Division of Obstetrics and Gynaecology
Karolinska University Hospital
Stockholm
Sweden

Olav Istre MD PhD
Department of Gynecology and Obstetrics
    Endoscopic Unit
Ullevaal University Hospital
Oslo
Norway

Eric Jauniaux MD PhD MRCOG
Professor in Obstetrics and Fetal Medicine at
    the Academic Department of Obstetrics and
    Gynaecology
University College London Medical School
    and Early Pregnancy Unit
Elizabeth Garrett Anderson Hospital
London
UK

Jemma Johns MRCOG
Academic Department of Obstetrics and
    Gynaecology
University College London Medical School
London
UK

Emma Kirk MBBS
Early Pregnancy, Gynaecological Ultrasound
    and MAS Unit
St George's, University of London
London
UK

Sven Nielsen MD PhD
Women's Clinic
Gothenburg
Sweden

Michael J Seckl BSc PhD MRCP
Gestational Trophoblastic Disease Unit
Department of Medical Oncology
Charing Cross and Hammersmith Hospitals
    Campus
Imperial College London
UK

Johanna Trinder MRCOG
Department of Obstetrics and Gynaecology
St. Michael's Hospital
Bristol
UK

Preface

For years the management of early pregnancy complications was very much the poor relation when training in gynaecology. In general the most junior doctor available was delegated to see the patient and perform any surgery, if indicated. Yet they are among the most common conditions seen by gynaecologists and cause a huge amount of anxiety and distress for patients.

The introduction of transvaginal ultrasonography, laparoscopic surgery and the rapid measurement of serum hCG levels has radically changed the face of early pregnancy management. More recently there has been an appreciation that less is perhaps more. Surgery has become less aggressive. Furthermore we now know that women do not have to undergo surgical intervention for miscarriage or ectopic pregnancy. It may be possible to adopt a watch and wait policy or use medical therapy.

Early pregnancy services have also become rationalized with standalone 'early pregnancy units'. These in turn have been organized in the UK into a society: The Association of Early Pregnancy Units. To work in such a unit requires experience with transvaginal ultrasonography and an understanding of the behaviour of serum hCG in both normal and abnormal early pregnancy. Such work is emotionally demanding. Understanding the management options available to women is important, we hope that this book helps to outline some of those options.

Tom Bourne
George Condous

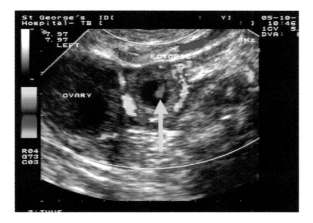

Figure 8.3 Viable tubal ectopic pregnancy; solid arrow points to fetal cardiac activity demonstrated with colour Doppler.

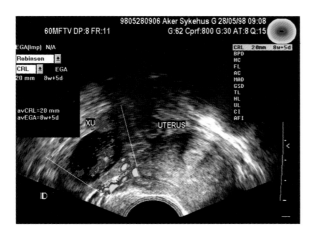

Figure 11.2 Transvaginal ultrasound of a live ectopic pregnancy at 8 weeks 5 days.

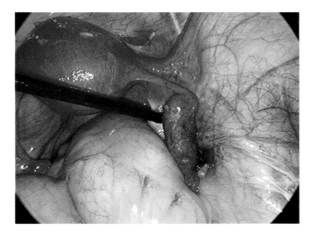

Figure 11.3 Laparoscopic view of an ampullary ectopic pregnancy.

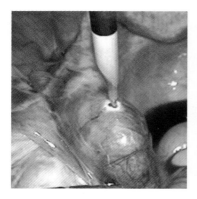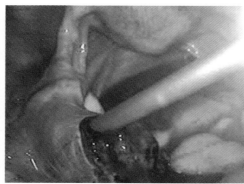

Figure 11.4 Laparoscopic salpingotomy in a left-sided ampullary ectopic pregnancy.

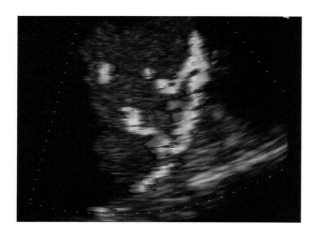

Figure 15.6 Endometrioma with vascular solid papillary projection on colour Doppler, consistent with endometrioid adenocarcinoma.

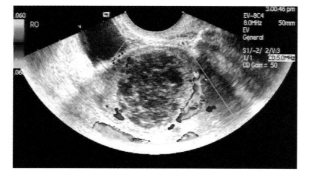

Figure 15.7 Haemorrhagic corpus luteum with a 'ring of fire' demonstrated using colour Doppler.

1

Setting up and running an Early Pregnancy Unit: space, staffing and equipment

Maha Alkatib

Introduction • Logistical requirements • Record keeping • Laboratory services • Emergency operating theatres • Information and protocols • Additional services • Conclusion • Practical points

INTRODUCTION

Early pregnancy complications represent a significant number of attendances both to primary care and hospital emergency (A&E) departments. Considering at least one in four pregnant women will have a miscarriage in the first trimester, and up to one in 50 will have an ectopic pregnancy, the rapid identification, management and aftercare of such women can clearly be seen to be of benefit to the woman's wellbeing as well as an effective use of resources.[1]

Traditionally, women would either attend a hospital emergency room or see their primary care physician if they were experiencing any bleeding or pain in the first trimester. Following an initial assessment with or without a vaginal examination, referral to the on-call gynaecologist would occur. Further assessment and vaginal examination would take place, and depending on experience, a further senior opinion would often be required before other investigations were arranged. Access to ultrasound facilities were often limited, resulting in admission of the woman until a scan was possible. Any serum investigations ordered could take more than 24 hours before a result

was obtained. Should surgery be necessary, a further wait on the emergency operating list could be expected resulting in prolonged fasting times until the operation was possible. A wholly unacceptable experience physically, mentally and financially.

As a consequence, in the United Kingdom, the Royal College of Obstetricians and Gynaecologists (RCOG) introduced a guideline recommending the setting up of a dedicated Early Pregnancy Unit (EPU) in all hospitals, to be accessible by other hospital departments, general practitioners (GPs) and women. This guideline stipulated that the facility should be available on a daily basis or during normal working hours as a minimum.[2] Benefits such as rapid diagnosis, creation of a sympathetic environment, prompt gynaecological input, accessible dedicated scanning facilities, reduced unnecessary admissions, reduced costs and preservation of women's dignity were achieved through such units.[1,3,4]

Setting up an EPU demands some basic resources for an effective, safe and efficient service to be achieved. This can be divided into logistical requirements, information and protocols, and additional services. For many years the management of early pregnancy complications was not seen as a high priority for gynaecologists – perhaps because it was perceived as not being as cutting edge as oncology or subfertility. However, the fact remains that complications in early pregnancy are common and are often the first contact a woman has with her local hospital. How well the problem is dealt with may dictate the woman's decision to book for delivery at that unit in her current or future pregnancies.

LOGISTICAL REQUIREMENTS

Location

A dedicated EPU area which is sign-posted in the hospital gives recognition to its existence and reduces an already raised level of anxiety in a woman trying to locate it. The EPU is usually located in the vicinity of the gynaecology outpatients department or the gynaecology ward in order to optimize availability of staff. Attempts to avoid locating it near the antenatal clinic should be made in order to reduce any distress experienced by women seeing ongoing pregnancies while waiting. Another option is to position the unit by the emergency room for ease of access for women coming through that route of referral.

The waiting area should have appropriate audio-visual facilities available – it is a walk-in service and women may have a significant wait before being seen. Toilet facilities that are easy to locate and within close proximity to the unit enable urine samples to be obtained discretely and quickly, as well ensuring an empty bladder prior to transvaginal sonography (TVS). Vending facilities should be avoided to optimize the chance of women being fasted should they require surgical intervention following their diagnosis.

Rooms

In certain units, a separate ultrasonographer is required to perform the TVS. In such circumstances a room that can be locked or screened from the door is necessary to accommodate the ultrasound machine and assessment. A separate room is then necessary for history taking and examination before and/or after the TVS – again, this requires a room that can be locked or has a screen from the door to guarantee privacy while the woman is changing and being examined. It is helpful to subdivide a single room with a curtain to give a woman privacy whilst changing. These rooms should be warm, welcoming and have good lighting for vaginal examinations. In other units, the nursing, midwifery or medical staff will have been trained in TVS in which case one room will suffice for all purposes. Depending on resources and funding, more than one scanning room can be running if the trained personnel are available.

Invariably, given the nature of the problems, emotional distress is regularly encountered. The clinical environment in the examination rooms is usually inhibiting and can increase any grief being experienced. It may also be that women wish to have some time to reflect and compose themselves before proceeding with any further management. The waiting area is not suitable for such women, and due to time constraints, the examination room cannot be used in this way. The availability of a counselling room with telephone access to allow calls to relatives or friends if necessary can be very valuable.

Staffing

There are different models for staffing an EPU. However it is the author's opinion that the person scanning the woman should also be able to explain the diagnosis and plan initial management. There must also be back up from a gynaecologist with a specific interest in the subject. The staff responsible for managing women must be proficient at ultrasonography and have a thorough knowledge of the behaviour of the serum hormones human chorionic gonadotrophin (hCG) and progesterone in pregnancy. Any gynaecologist supervizing the unit must be able to scan, perform laparoscopic surgery and should be conversant with the conservative management of early pregnancy complications.

Receptionist – will have access to the hospital appointments system in order to register every episode of attendance and arrange follow-up appointments accordingly. They will be the point of all enquiries from GPs, A&E and women waiting. They can also distribute information leaflets at the time of women registering, thereby ensuring all women have a basic knowledge of what to expect while in the EPU.

Nurse/Midwife Practitioner – such individuals should be experienced either in gynaecology nursing or midwifery, with a solid background of dealing with early pregnancy complications. They should be trained to perform TVS; this reduces the number of individuals the woman encounters before a diagnosis is reached, and this may well be the only person she will have to see in the EPU if conservative management is appropriate. In many cases an effective EPU can be nurse run. However there must be effective medical input for interventions. Ultrasonographers trained to the standards of the Royal College of Radiologists or other national body requirements with regards to TVS and transabdominal scanning (TAS) and reporting in a standardized format will also play a part in diagnostics.[5]

Gynaecologist – Senior House Officer (SHO) or junior resident level as a minimum requirement, and who is available when needed. This can either be the SHO on-call or one who is timetabled to be in the EPU for a particular session in order to obtain exposure and training in early pregnancy complications and TVS. There should be a senior gynaecologist available to make decisions about the management of pregnancies of unknown location (PULs) and ectopic pregnancy. Ideally this should be a named lead consultant who takes overall responsibility for the unit.

Chaperone – the RCOG stipulates the need for a chaperone during any form of examination of women by both genders.[6] This can be done by a healthcare assistant or less experienced nursing staff.

Women's counsellor – access to such an individual is valuable given the proven psychological sequelae of early pregnancy loss.[7] Although their presence on a day-to-day basis is not absolutely necessary, having an appointment-based system that is accessible by women should they wish to speak to someone is helpful.

Communication – it is important that there is good communication within the team. Individual cases will be discussed on a daily basis; however, there should also be a weekly multidisciplinary team (MDT) meeting to discuss cases and risk events. This meeting should be minuted and action points made and reviewed the following week.

Equipment

Ultrasound machine – the ability to perform transvaginal and transabdominal scans is necessary. TVS has been found to be acceptable by women having an elective pregnancy scan.[8] If appropriate reassurance is given in the information leaflet and consultation prior to the scan, women are usually reassured that this will not affect their pregnancy in any way. The transvaginal probe should have a frequency range of 5–7.5 MHz enabling sufficient resolution to identify ectopic pregnancies and early intrauterine pregnancies as early as possible. A 3.5-MHz transabdominal probe is sufficient for assessment of second-trimester pregnancies and women declining TVS. The ability to take hard copies of all images is a requirement whether through a printer or digitally – a photograph can then be given to the woman if requested. Any additional features such as 3D/4D or colour Doppler imaging are of little value in the day-to-day running of an EPU and are usually limited to research purposes. The majority of the work in an EPU can be carried out on what are now small portable machines at the low end of the spectrum in terms of cost.

Refrigeration/drugs cabinet – Anti-D immunoglobulin and ergometrine require storage at around 0°C and away from direct sunlight. To enable a comprehensive service being offered, having Anti-D available if the rhesus status is known ensures completion of management of women and avoids the involvement of additional services.[9] Occasionally, women will present or subsequently develop much heavier bleeding while waiting which may require the administration of ergometrine while stabilizing them. Immediate access reduces blood loss and brings control to the situation sooner.

Basic analgesia, antibiotics, prostaglandins and antiemetics that are routinely used in the management of early pregnancy complications should be readily available. If such medications can be offered to the patient at the point of discharge, this minimizes time spent in the hospital, potentially benefits a woman's mental wellbeing as well as reducing the workload on the main pharmacy.

RECORD KEEPING

The patient administration system (PAS) will enable appointments and events to be logged but does not archive any greater detail. History, examination and scan findings need to be documented and archived in the woman's patient notes or on a database that is backed up by the hospital computer servers. Restricted password-based access to preserve patient confidentiality, and unique identifying numbers for each woman are essential when relying on a computer-based archive. The advantages of a computer database include instant access to previous episodes, instant updating of events at any terminal by authorized individuals, archiving of digital images for each visit if image-capturing facilities exist and the ability to perform audit and research on a vast database of information. Such software packages exist and can be married up to the hospital computer network for access to the information as simply as when accessing blood results.

LABORATORY SERVICES

Access to haematology, blood bank and biochemistry on an urgent and routine basis is a basic requirement. Haemoglobin levels in women with significant bleeding/suspected ectopic pregnancies/preoperatively is usually required, as well as a knowledge of their rhesus status in the event of them requiring Anti-D if they meet the criteria for having it.[9] Sickle cell status in the Afro-Caribbean population is mandatory if surgery is necessary.

Serum hCG levels (World Health Organization, Third International Reference 57/537) are pivotal in the management of pregnancies of unknown location and suspected ectopic pregnancies. Although the RCOG recommends that results should be available within 24 hours in practice this is not good enough. The results must be available on the same working day or within 4 hours in order that a women can have a management plan put in place.[2] Such an approach may reduce unnecessary delay and morbidity in women who are believed to have a high index of suspicion for ectopic pregnancy. A patient having had her blood taken in the morning can be rung at home with results and instructions given regarding management, including the possibility of coming back to hospital.

Microbiology services for microscopy, culture and sensitivity of urine samples and high vaginal swabs aid in diagnosis and management of coinciding ailments women may be experiencing.

EMERGENCY OPERATING THEATRES

The EPU needs to be located in a hospital where emergency operating facilities are on site. These usually require that the woman is admitted as an inpatient before they can be placed on the list. The problem with such lists is that they are accessible by all surgical specialities and cases are performed in order of priority and timing. Ways of reducing the need for this system will be discussed later. Some units may have beds on the gynaecology ward specifically for women requiring emergency gynaecology surgery. This ensures that they are in the correct ward rather than a non-gynaecological ward as a result of bed availability, and waiting for a bed is not delayed.

INFORMATION AND PROTOCOLS

The majority of EPUs will be nurse-run, requiring very little input from a gynaecologist if appropriate protocols are created and adhered to. With the current emphasis on evidence-based practice and clinical governance to optimize patient care and reduce adverse events and risk incidents, clearly defined protocols are a prerequisite to the successful functioning of an EPU. This guarantees a consistent approach to all problems and becomes independent of staff turnover. Individual protocols for all early pregnancy complications should be compiled into a file and placed in every assessment room for reference. These protocols will include fine details such as dosage regimens and timings between visits. Protocols relating to referral criteria, initial assessment, management of miscarriage, ectopic pregnancies, pregnancies of unknown location, gestational trophoblastic disease and hyperemesis gravidarum should be developed and made available to all members of the early pregnancy team. The evidence for each protocol is stated at the end of each section and the date of compilation also stipulated. Protocols should be revised on an annual basis according to current NHS recommendations. A suggested series of protocols will be offered in the following chapters.

Women attending EPUs will not be able to absorb all the information relayed to them verbally and so rely upon written information to supplement and remind them of discussions that took place during the consultation. This written information also answers questions that may not have been considered at the time. Each type of early pregnancy problem has advice specific and appropriate to it that needs to be passed on to women. Given this, the creation of patient information leaflets for each early pregnancy complication can ensure women are informed of the underlying cause, what to expect now and what the future holds for them. This information can also be placed on the unit or hospital website for reference. Clear warning of symptoms/signs that require urgent action should also be found in such leaflets. The language should be clear, must avoid using medical jargon and explain medical terms clearly when necessary. Diagrams may help in explaining the problem more clearly, e.g. ectopic pregnancy. Contact numbers for the unit and numbers to call in the event of an emergency should be clearly outlined in every leaflet, especially those pertaining to pregnancies of unknown location or medical management of ectopic pregnancies. Women should know exactly who to contact and where to go in any given 24-hour period. Most hospital leaflets are now vetted and approved by a dedicated patient information services department. This should be done in consultation with them for clinical governance purposes.

ADDITIONAL SERVICES

The following are suggestions for optimizing the service further than the basic requirements, thereby improving the woman's experience and making efficient use of hospital resources.

Self-referral service

The majority of EPUs employ an appointment-based system – the primary care physician contacts the unit to refer the woman and they are given an appointment to be seen within the next 24 hours. Some women who have used the unit before may call for advice and can be given an appointment to be seen if deemed necessary. Employing a self-referral or walk-in service similar to an emergency room set-up has been employed by a few units. Although this does increase the numbers attending on a daily basis, the system is not abused and has been found to be of benefit to women psychologically. Women eligible for this walk-in service include bleeding and/or pain in the first trimester of pregnancy with a confirmed positive urinary hCG, a history of previous miscarriages resulting in maternal anxiety, history of previous ectopic pregnancy, and pregnancy following sterilization or insertion of an intrauterine contraceptive device. Women who are uncertain of their dates and wish to confirm gestational age, in order for GPs to know when to arrange nuchal scans, are also seen in such units. Such women will be given an appointment to be seen within the week. In our unit in a busy teaching hospital, as many as 25 women per day can be seen in a 4-hour period by two trained nurse/midwife sonographers with no woman being turned away during the opening hours of the unit. A positive urinary hCG must be confirmed before a patient is seen.

Emergency gynaecology operating list

Creating a dedicated emergency gynaecology operating list at regular intervals during the week can dramatically reduce the number of inpatient beds used while waiting for cases to be performed on the emergency operating lists in otherwise stable women. This can be run as a day-case list for stable women so they do not require a bed preoperatively and can leave 2 to 4 hours postoperatively if escorted. There should be a named consultant covering or performing the list with a named registrar or resident also allocated to it. All surgical evacuations of the uterus after miscarriage and cases with stable ectopic pregnancies suitable for laparoscopic salpingectomy/salpingotomy can be performed on these lists. Day surgery for ectopic pregnancy is safe. In our unit we run lists on a Monday, Wednesday and Friday, and the majority of ectopic pregnancies can be fitted into this schedule. They do not all need to undergo surgery on the day of diagnosis. This offers an ideal training opportunity under senior supervision during normal working hours. This reduces the number of procedures performed out-of-hours thereby reducing on-call workloads and laparotomies due to laparoscopic inexperience/equipment being unavailable.

Chlamydia screening

The prevalence of *Chlamydia* has increased in the population, as has the incidence of ectopic pregnancies.[11] Screening in women of reproductive age to reduce long term fertility complications and ectopic pregnancy rates from subclinical chlamydial infection is simple to perform and should be done opportunistically in such a setting with permission being sought from women prior to performing the test. A low vaginal swab performed by the woman herself with clear instructions has a sensitivity of 90% with the newer swab mediums.[12]

CONCLUSION

EPUs should be an integral part of all Departments of Obstetrics and Gynaecology, functioning alongside emergency departments in facilitating the rapid and sensitive management of women with early pregnancy complications. Having a dedicated ultrasound-based unit guarantees continuity of care and optimizes the management of pregnancies of unknown location and ectopic pregnancies. The location, setting and staffing of the unit is instrumental in the functioning of such a unit and has been covered in this chapter. Ensuring correct and clear information and protocols are available reduces the amount of human error that can result in their absence. The psychological wellbeing of a woman during her experience in hospital is an important factor not to be neglected when thinking about running an EPU. Having appropriate counselling facilities and staff trained in recognizing signs of psychological morbidity that may require further surveillance can prevent any adverse outcomes for the woman.

PRACTICAL POINTS

1. EPUs should be an integral part of the Obstetrics and Gynaecology Unit in any hospital.
2. EPUs require their own dedicated and trained staff members in an environment that attempts to reduce women's anxiety and preserve their dignity.
3. Transvaginal ultrasound should be the first mode of assessment vs transabdominal.
4. Clear record keeping and image archiving is essential with the use of computer software being of added benefit.
5. Serum hCG assays should be possible within 4–6 hours of the sample being received by the lab.
6. Clear protocols that are regularly updated should be available in every examination room.
7. Women should be kept well informed throughout their visit to the EPU and have this supplemented with information leaflets.
8. Developing a walk-in service and dedicated emergency gynaecology day surgery operating lists can improve a woman's experience as well as being cost-effective.

REFERENCES

1. Bigrigg MA, Read MD. Management of women referred to early pregnancy assessment unit: care and cost effectiveness. BMJ 1998; 316:1324–5.

2. Royal College of Obstetricians and Gynaecologists. The management of early pregnancy loss. Guideline No. 25. RCOG Press, London, 2000.

3. Bradley E, Hamilton-Fairley D. Managing miscarriage in early pregnancy assessment units. Hosp Med 1998; 59(6):451–6.

4. Walker JJ, Shillito J. Early pregnancy assessment units: service and organisational aspects. In: Grudzinskas JG, O'Brien PMS (eds). Problems in early pregnancy: advances in diagnosis and management. London: RCOG Press, 1997; 160–73.

5. Guidance on ultrasound procedures in early pregnancy. Report of the RCR & RCOG Working Party. London, 1995.

6. Royal College of Obstetricians and Gynaecologists. Gynaecological Examinations: Guidelines for specialist practice. RCOG Press, London, 2002.

7. Seibel M, Graves WL. The psychological implications of spontaneous abortions. J Reprod Med 1980; 25(4): 161–5.

8. Braithwaite JM, Economides DL. Acceptability of patients of transvaginal sonography in the elective assessment of the first-trimester fetus. Ultrasound Obstet Gynecol 1997; 9(2):91–3.

9. Royal College of Obstetricians and Gynaecologists. Use of Anti-D immunoglobulin for Rh prophylaxis. RCOG Press, London, 2002.

10. Trends in sexually transmitted infections in the United Kingdom, 1990–1999. New episodes seen at genito-urinary medicine clinics: PHLS (England, Wales & Northern Ireland), DHSS & PS (Northern Ireland) and the Scottish ISD(D)5 Collaborative Group (ISD, SCIEH and MSSVD). London: Public Health Laboratory Service; December 2000.

11. Garrow SC, Smith DW, Harnett GB. The diagnosis of chlamydia, gonorrhoea, and trichomonas infections by self obtained low vaginal swabs, in remote northern Australian clinical practice. Sex Transmit Infect 2002; 78(4):278–81.

2

Normal findings and development in early pregnancy

Jemma Johns and Eric Jauniaux

Introduction • History taking • Normal human development • Identification of fetal structural anomalies in the first trimester • Practical points

INTRODUCTION

The advent of high-resolution transvaginal ultrasound has revolutionized our understanding of the development of normal early human pregnancy. Knowledge of the ultrasound appearances in normal early pregnancy and a good understanding of the pitfalls, especially in the emergency setting, is essential for the accurate diagnosis and management of early pregnancy problems. The first demonstration of an early intrauterine pregnancy by means of a transvaginal ultrasound scan (TVS) was reported in 1967.[1] Since then, dramatic improvements have occurred and the development of high-resolution ultrasound imaging has enabled the anatomy and physiology of the human fetus to be studied in vivo from as early as the 3rd week postimplantation onwards.

As we have seen in Chapter 1, the introduction of early pregnancy units (EPUs) into many hospitals has resulted in significant changes, both in the management of early pregnancy, and also in the training and development of scanning skills for junior doctors, nurses and midwives. On the one hand, training of junior staff has become more structured and better supervised. On the other, reductions in junior doctors' hours and less time allocated to developing special skills may have left many juniors with limited experience of early pregnancy scanning. The development of highly sensitive urinary human chorionic gonadotrophin (hCG) assays and a greater awareness of early pregnancy ultrasound amongst healthcare professionals and women alike has resulted in ever earlier presentation. This has led to an increase in the number of non-diagnostic scans and as a result an increase in the requirement for repeat assessments to determine both pregnancy location and viability. This chapter aims to describe the 'normal ultrasound appearance' of early human pregnancy and also to tackle some of the common pitfalls that can occur when the findings are not as expected.

HISTORY TAKING

Before performing an ultrasound in early pregnancy, there are essential pieces of information from the history that will assist in preparation for what 'should' be seen. These are presented below and may seem obvious but are commonly overlooked in the desire to perform a scan and make a quick diagnosis.

Last menstrual period (LMP) and cycle length

Knowledge of the first day of the LMP and the cycle length in any individual can alter the

Table 2.1. Correction of dates for cycle length	
Cycle length (day 1 to day 1) e.g.	Number of days difference in gestation (based on typical obstetric calendar)
21 days	+7
28 days	0
35 days	−7
40 days	−12

expected gestation and therefore the ultrasound findings considerably and may make the difference between seeing an early pregnancy and having a non-diagnostic scan that necessitates follow-up. Correction for cycle length is therefore important if the length deviates by 7 or more days from a 28-day cycle (Table 2.1).

It should be remembered, however, that recall of the exact LMP also varies considerably but probably has little impact in clinical practice. Pregnancies that are conceived whilst on the oral contraceptive pill can be dated reasonably accurately from the date of the last withdrawal bleed,[2] however dating of conceptions from non-bleed forms of contraception will rely on detailed history taking (likely time of conception, date of positive pregnancy test) and ultrasound findings.

Conception history

Knowledge of details surrounding the conception can have a considerable impact on the ultrasound findings. As mentioned above, the knowledge that the pregnancy was conceived on the oral contraceptive pill may affect the dating of the pregnancy. In addition, conception with an intrauterine contraceptive device (IUCD) or system (IUS) will increase the index of suspicion of an ectopic pregnancy.

It is important to be aware whether this was a spontaneous pregnancy or one achieved by assisted reproduction techniques (ART). Many women may not be able to provide an accurate LMP but will be able to state the exact date of their intrauterine insemination (IUI) or embryo

transfer (ET), assisting in the dating process. When performing an ultrasound on a woman after ART it is essential to be aware of the possible increased risk of ectopic pregnancy,[3] heterotopic pregnancy[4] and the likely presence of multiple ovarian cysts, if cycles were stimulated. It may also be relevant to enquire about past gynaecological history as the presence of uterine fibroids or previous surgery may alter the ultrasound findings.

Pregnancy tests

The timing of the positive pregnancy test may also help determine the dates of the pregnancy if there is uncertainty surrounding the LMP. Often several tests will have been performed and this information can be very useful when ultrasound findings are not as expected.

Endocrinological tests

In most cases of early pregnancy assessment, hCG and progesterone assays are not required unless the location of the pregnancy is in doubt. Knowledge of the 'normal' increases in hCG levels in early pregnancy are useful as a guide after a non-diagnostic ultrasound of pregnancy of unknown location, provided they are combined with other features such as clinical symptoms, other ultrasound findings and progesterone results.[5,6] The hCG 'doubling time' is used as a guide to the viability and location of an early gestation, although it must be remembered that in very early pregnancy the doubling time both for intrauterine and ectopic pregnancies can be similar and also shorter than later in the first trimester.[7] Further discussion of serum biochemistry in normal and abnormal early pregnancy is outside the scope of this chapter and is discussed in detail later in the book, and we have provided the normal ranges for gestation as a rough guide only. The following descriptions of TVS findings and hCG levels are based on a spontaneous pregnancy in a 28-day cycle and gestations represent the postmenstrual age rather than the postconception age. The chapter concentrates on the first 14 weeks of pregnancy.

Table 2.2. Relationship between transvaginal ultrasound findings and hCG levels

Gestational age (weeks)	Embryological features (TVS)	Anatomical landmarks	hCG[8] (IU/L)
4	Trophoblastic ring Gestation sac ~ 2 mm		600–1000
5	Secondary yolk sac Gestation sac 8–10 mm Embryo 1–2 mm[9] ± FHB		6000–10 000
6	Embryo 4–9 mm[9] Gestation sac 16–40 mm FHB +		>10 000
7	Embryo 10–15 mm[9] Gestation sac FHB +	Rhombencephalon ± Upper limb buds	>10 000
8	Embryo 16–22 mm[9] Gestation sac ± Fetal movements	± Mid gut herniation ± Fetal stomach	>10 000
9	Embryo 23–30 mm[9]	Mid gut herniation ± Fetal stomach	10 000
10	Embryo 31–40 mm[9]	Mid gut herniation ± Fetal bladder Clavicle/femur/skull base mineralisation ± Fetal stomach	>10 000
11	Embryo 41–52 mm[9]	± Mid gut herniation ± Fetal bladder Fetal stomach Cranial vault mineralisation	>10 000
12	Embryo 53–66 mm[9] Obliteration of SYS & ECC	Fetal bladder Cranial vault mineralisation Complete retraction of mid gut herniation 4-chamber cardiac view	>10 000

The ultrasound scan

Before embarking on an ultrasound it helps to ask yourself a few questions:

1. What am I trying to find out by performing a scan?
2. Does the scan need to be performed now or can it wait?
3. Will the scan change my management?
4. What type of scan do I need to perform i.e. transvaginal or transabdominal?

In the emergency setting, your decision to perform an ultrasound may not always be correct and we have all been in the situation when we wish that we had not! Always be sure that you are competent to perform the scan that is required and that it will alter the management plan for the woman. Be prepared to act upon the scan result. In most situations in the early pregnancy setting, a transvaginal rather than transabdominal approach is preferred. Occasionally, a transabdominal scan (TAS) is required to assess intra-abdominal pathology such as large ovarian cysts, fibroids or ascites. TVS does not require a full bladder (which can be an advantage in someone who is nil-by-mouth or vomiting). Remember, the first scan in women who present to an EPU should be performed transvaginally. This accurately dates the pregnancy, confirms the viability and locates the pregnancy at earlier gestations compared to the transabdominal route.

NORMAL HUMAN DEVELOPMENT (TABLE 2.2)

Week 4

Ultrasound scanning at this very early gestation can be difficult because of the reasons stated above. Often the only ultrasound feature visible is a thickening of the endometrium and the presence of a corpus luteum cyst. The deciduo–placental interface and the exocoelomic cavity (ECC) are the first sonographic evidence of a pregnancy that can be visualized with TVS from around 4^{+4}–4^{+6} menstrual weeks (32–34 days) when they reach together a size of 2 to 4 mm (visible at approximately 5 weeks or 10 mm on TAS). They appear as an echogenic or 'trophoblastic' ring, consisting of the decidua capsularis and the chorion laeve, which is eccentrically placed within the endometrium (i.e. to one side of the midline of the endometrium, within the endometrium), with a sonolucent centre representing the ECC (Figure 2.1). The corresponding hCG level at this stage would be 600–1000 IU/L.[8] The location of the intrauterine sac is important and should not be mistaken for the collection of fluid between the two layers of endometrium (sometimes seen in ectopic pregnancies). This is known confusingly as a 'pseudosac' and the term should no longer be used in modern practice. This historic term was based on TAS findings and with the use of high-resolution TVS probes, we believe that those performing a scan should be able to differentiate between a true intrauterine sac and fluid in the cavity.

Week 5

In normal intrauterine pregnancies between the 5th and 6th weeks, the gestation sac grows at a rate of approximately 1 mm/day in mean diameter.[10,11] The hCG at this gestation should be approximately 6000–10 000 IU/L.[8] The first structure to be seen inside the chorionic sac, before the embryo itself, is the secondary yolk sac (SYS) which can be observed from the beginning of the 5th week of gestation or when the gestational sac reaches 10 mm in diameter (Figure 2.2).[8,12] The SYS can be seen as a spherical structure with a bright outline and a sonolucent centre. The visualization of the

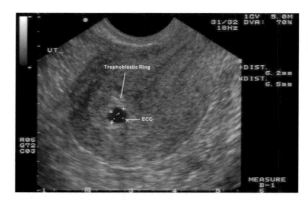

Figure 2.1 Trophoblastic ring at 4 weeks' gestation consisting of decidua capsularis, chorion laeve and exocoelomic cavity (ECC).

secondary yolk sac is a reassuring finding, confirming the presence of an intrauterine pregnancy. It should never be forgotten however that the incidence of heterotopic pregnancy is increasing (1% in the IVF population[4]) and a history of ART, clinical symptoms not in keeping with an intrauterine pregnancy, or additional ultrasound findings such as an adnexal mass or significant free fluid in the pouch of Douglas should arouse suspicion and trigger a search for a heterotopic pregnancy. Measurement of the crown–rump length (CRL) is still the main reference for the assessment of gestational age in early pregnancy.[13] Because TVS provides superior resolution and more accurate identification of the embryonic structures than abdominal ultrasound, new charts have been developed for the period of gestation before 7 weeks.[9] The fetal pole can be visualized within the ECC as a thickening of the wall of the SYS and is located closest to the uterine wall (Figure 2.3). The fetal pole should be visualized on TVS from the end of the 5th week where it will be approximately 2 mm.

Fetal cardiac activity is the earliest proof of a viable pregnancy and it has been documented in utero by TVS as early as 26 days postconceptional age,[14] approximately at the time when the heart tube starts to beat.[15] Theoretically, cardiac activity should always be evident when the embryo is over 2 mm.[16] However, in around

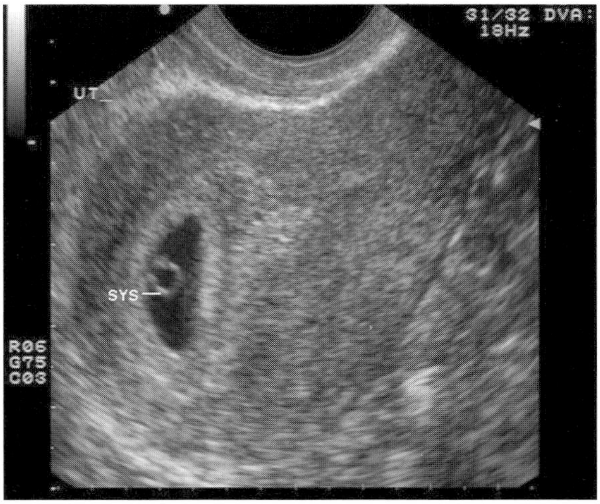

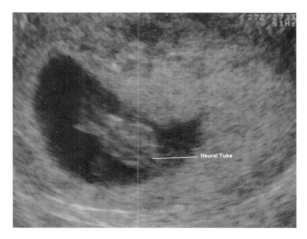

Figure 2.4 Neural tube at 8 weeks' gestation.

Figure 2.2 Five-week pregnancy with secondary yolk sac (SYS).

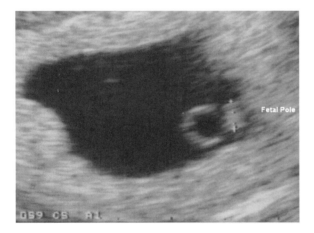

Figure 2.3 Six-week gestation with SYS and fetal pole.

Week 6

During the sixth week, the embryo grows rapidly. The amniotic membrane becomes visible as the amniotic cavity expands and the embryo appears distinct from the SYS. The CRL ranges between 4–9 mm and the gestational sac measures approximately 16–40 mm.[9] Fetal heart activity should be clearly visible. The hCG will now remain above 10 000 IU/L for the duration of the first trimester.[8] The first anatomical feature to become visible is at this stage and is the primitive neural tube. This can be seen as two parallel lines with a hypoechoic region running down the centre (Figure 2.4).[24]

Week 7

By the seventh week, the amniotic membrane and cavity are more distinct and the SYS can be seen to be suspended in the ECC. The fetal pole measures 10–15 mm[9] and shows definite polarity with the fetal head clearly visible. The fetal head contains a large sonolucent area representing the rhombencephalon or hindbrain (Figure 2.5).[25] This area will later become the fourth ventricle. The upper limb buds may also be visible as small paddles at this gestation and the umbilical cord can be visualized.

5–10% of embryos between 2 and 4 mm it can not be demonstrated, although the corresponding pregnancies will have a normal outcome.[17,18] From 5 to 9 weeks of gestation there is a rapid increase in the mean heart rate from 110 to 175 beats per minutes (bpm). The heart rate then gradually decreases to around 160 to 170 bpm.[15,19–23] Measurements of fetal heart rates in early pregnancy have limited prognostic value and should not be measured in the routine assessment of early pregnancy.

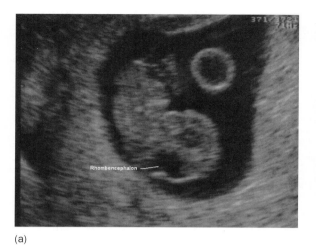

(a)

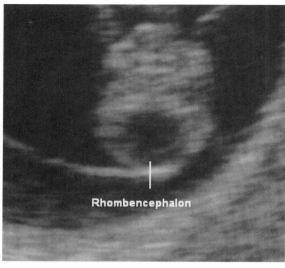

(b)

Figure 2.5 (a) Sagittal view of rhombencephalon at 7 weeks' gestation. (b) Axial view of rhombencephalon at 7 weeks' gestation.

Week 8

The fetal pole ranges from 16–22 mm in week eight, fetal movements may become apparent and the upper and lower limb buds become clearer.[26] The physiological mid-gut herniation can be seen from the middle of the eighth week (Figure 2.6) and the fetal stomach may also be visualized.[27]. The vessels of the cord can also be visualized. There are now several sonolucent areas within the fetal brain representing the prosencephalon (forebrain), mesencephalon (midbrain) and the rhombencephalon (Figure 2.7). The cerebellum and choroid plexus can also be visualized during week eight by TVS.[25]

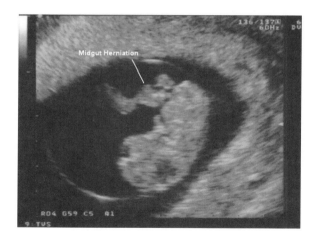

Figure 2.6 Physiological mid-gut herniation at 8 weeks' gestation.

Weeks 9–12

During this time the fetus and membranes develop rapidly. The amniotic cavity expands as the fetal metanephros starts to function and produce urine which is passed into the amniotic cavity.[28] Subsequently, with the accumulation of this fluid the amniotic membrane moves towards the fetal plate of the placenta (Figure 2.8), and the ECC, along with the degenerating SYS will almost entirely disappear by 12–13

weeks of gestation. The fetal bladder can be visualized from 10 weeks and should be visible in all cases by the end of the 12th week.[29] The CRL ranges from 23 mm at 9 weeks to 66 mm at the end of 12 weeks (Table 2.2).[9] The fetal stomach should be visible in all cases by 11 weeks and the retraction of the mid-gut herni-

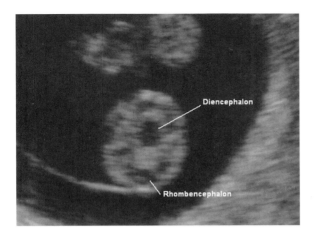

Figure 2.7 Prosencephalon and rhombencephalon at 8 weeks' gestation.

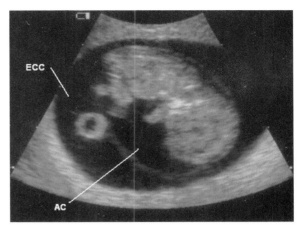

Figure 2.8 The enlarging amniotic cavity (AC) at 9 weeks' gestation.

ation is complete by the end of the 12th week.[27] Bone mineralization commences in the clavicle and femur and will be visible in the cranial vault by 10 weeks' gestation.[29] The limbs will develop distinct long bones and digits will become visible. It should also be possible to determine cardiac situs, and a four-chamber view in the majority of fetuses by 12 weeks' gestation.[30] The optimal time in the first trimester to perform transvaginal fetal echocardiography appears to be between 13 and 14 weeks.[31]

IDENTIFICATION OF FETAL STRUCTURAL ANOMALIES IN THE FIRST TRIMESTER

A detailed discussion of screening for fetal abnormalities and aneuploidy is outside the scope of this chapter and is generally not within the remit of the EPU or first trimester scan. An awareness of major developmental landmarks is important however, as many anomalies can be identified in the first trimester allowing early referral and management. The ability to recognize abnormalities and be able to discuss them with the parents will become more important as patient awareness and demand for earlier

diagnosis inevitably increases. Clearly, many anomalies will not be apparent in the first trimester and first trimester anomaly scanning will not replace the second trimester anatomy scan. However, the widespread introduction of Down syndrome screening, requiring accurate dating, with nuchal translucency and nasal bone assessment at the 10–14 week scan has resulted in many more anomalies being detectable in the first trimester.[32] It must be kept in mind that a proportion of such anomalies will result in spontaneous miscarriage, before assessment is carried out, and the emotional and financial burden of 'routine' anatomy scanning in the first trimester have yet to be adequately assessed.

In a meta-analysis of all studies examining the 'first-trimester anatomy scan', the overall detection rate for fetal abnormalities in the first trimester was 44%.[38] An overview of the detection rates for the different organ systems in the first trimester can be found in Table 2.3. The majority can be seen to be major abnormalities of the CNS (anencephaly (Figure 2.9), holoprosencephaly (Figure 2.10), encephalocele), and the gastrointestinal tract, in particular exomphalos (Figure 2.11).

Table 2.3. Detection rate of specific anomalies at the early pregnancy scan

Anomaly	Cases	Diagnosed (%)
Central nervous system	52/82	67%
Cardiovascular	10/46	22%
Urinary	33/76	43%
Skeletal	20/78	26%
Respiratory tract	0/3	0%
Gastrointestinal tract	23/37	62%
Other	9/12	75%
Total	147/334	44%

Reproduced by kind permission of Dr B Weisz.[38]

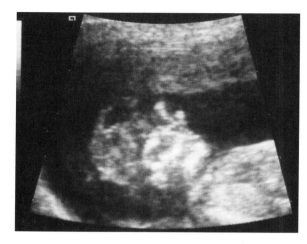

Figure 2.10 Holoprosencephaly at 12 weeks' gestation.

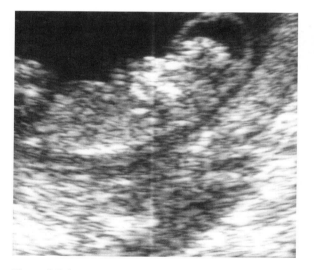

Figure 2.9 Acrania at 12 weeks' gestation.

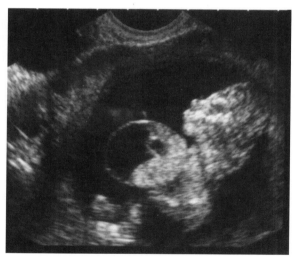

Figure 2.11 Omphalocele at 12 weeks' gestation.

There is good evidence that the use of TVS has improved our ability to identify structural abnormalities in the first trimester, that it is more sensitive than the transabdominal approach[33–35] and that a comprehensive fetal anatomical survey is possible with TVS in the first trimester.[36] A combination of the two approaches results in an even higher sensitivity.[37] We believe that in the future, more congenital anomalies will be diagnosed at earlier gestations in the first trimester – whether this will benefit women remains to be seen.

PRACTICAL POINTS

1. Apart from the result of a diagnostic test such as ultrasound, post-test odds of finding pathology are influenced by the prior odds, which in turn, are determined by the woman's clinical symptoms.
2. Therefore LMP, conception and contraceptive history are all important factors to consider prior to performing an ultrasound in early pregnancy.
3. This is highlighted in women who undergo ART and as a result have a heterotopic ectopic pregnancy rate as high as 1%.
4. When performing a scan in the EPU, the transvaginal is far superior to the transabdominal approach.
5. TVS in the first trimester confirms gestational age and viability of a pregnancy, but most importantly defines the location.
6. The first ultrasonographic finding in normal pregnancy is visualized at 4^{+4}–4^{+6} weeks – an echogenic ring, eccentrically placed within the endometrial cavity.
7. The fetal pole should be seen by the end of the 5th week of gestation.
8. Fetal cardiac activity is seen as early as 5^{+5} weeks gestation.
9. Remember 5–10% of embryos between 2 and 4 mm do not have fetal cardiac activity on TVS, but go on to have a normal outcome. Therefore if there is ANY doubt about the viabilty of a fetus, repeat the scan in 1 week.
10. Measuring fetal heart rates in the first trimester should only be done in the setting of clinical research.
11. First-trimester anomaly scans will not replace the second-trimester anatomy scan.

REFERENCES

1. Kratochwill E, Eisenhut L. Der fruheste nachweis der fatalen herzaction durch ultrascall. Geburtsh Frauenheik 1967; 27:176–80.
2. Waldenstrom U, Axelsson O, Nilsson S. Sonographic dating of pregnancies conceived after contraceptive pill therapy. Ultrasound Obstet Gynecol 1993; 3:23–25.
3. Barlow DH. Short- and long-term risks for women having IVF – what is the evidence? Hum Fertil 1999; 2:102–6.
4. Rizk B, Tan SL, Morcos S, et al. Heterotopic pregnancies after in vitro fertilization and embryo transfer. Am J Obstet Gynecol 1991; 164:161–64.
5. Banerjee S, Aslam N, Zosmer N, Woelfer B, Jurkovic D. The expectant management of women with early pregnancy of unknown location. Ultrasound Obstet Gynaecol 1999; 14:231–36.
6. Condous G, Okaro E, Khalid A, et al. The use of a new logistic regression model for predicting the outcome of pregnancies of unknown location. Hum Reprod 2004; 19:1900–10.
7. Check JH, Weiss RM, Lurie D. Analysis of serum human chorionic gonadotrophin levels in normal singleton, multiple and abnormal pregnancies. Hum Reprod 1992; 7:1176–80.
8. Bree LR, Marn CS. Transvaginal sonography in the first trimester: embryology, anatomy and hCG correlation. Semin Ultrasound CT MR 1990; 11:12–21.
9. Hadlock FP, Shah YP, Kanon DS, Lindsey JV. Fetal crown–rump length: re-evaluation of relation to menstrual age (5–18 weeks) with high resolution real time US. Radiology 1992; 182:501–5.
10. Nyberg DA, Mack LA, Laing FC, Patten RM. Distinguishing normal from abnormal gestational sac growth in early pregnancy. J Ultrasound Med 1987; 6:23–27.
11. Jauniaux ER, Jurkovic D. The role of ultrasound in abnormal early pregnancy. In: Grudzinskas JG, O'Brien PMS, eds. Problems in Early Pregnancy Advances in Diagnosis and Management. London: RCOG Press, 1997; 137.
12. Jauniaux E, Jurkovic D, Henriet Y, Rodesch F, Hustin J. Development of the secondary human yolk sac: correlation of sonographic and anatomic features. Hum Reprod 1991; 6:1160–6.
13. Robinson HP, Fleming JEE. A critical evaluation of sonar 'crown–rump length' measurements. Br J Obstet Gynecol 1975; 82:702–10.
14. Howe RS, Isaacson KJ, Albert JL, Coutifaris CB. Embryonic heart rate in human pregnancy. J Ultrasound Med 1991; 10:367–71.
15. Tezuka N, Sato S, Kanasugi H, Hiroi M. Embryonic heart rates: development in early first trimester and

clinical evaluation. Gynecol Obstet Invest 1991; 32:210–12.

16. Levi CS, Lyons EA, Zheng XH, Lindsay DJ, Holt SC. Endovaginal US: demonstration of cardiac activity in embryos of less than 5.0 mm in crown–rump length. Radiology 1990; 176:71–4.

17. Goldstein SR. Significance of cardiac activity on endovaginal ultrasound in very early embryos. Obstet Gynecol 1992; 80:670–2.

18. Brown DL, Emerson DS, Felker RE, Cartier MS, Smith WC. Diagnosis of early embryonic demise by endovaginal sonography. J Ultrasound Med 1990; 9:631–6.

19. Stefos TI, Lolis DE, Sotiriadis AJ, Ziakas GV. Embryonic heart rate in early pregnancy. J Clin Ultrasound 1998; 26:33–6.

20. van Heeswijk M, Nijhuis JG, Hollanders HM. Fetal heart rate in early pregnancy. Early Hum Dev 1990; 22:151–6.

21. Achiron R, Tadmore O, Mashiach S. Heart rate as a predictor of first-trimester spontaneous abortion after ultrasound proven viability. Obstet Gynecol 1991; 78:330–4.

22. Coulam CB, Britten S, Soenksen DM. Early (34–56 days from last menstrual period) ultrasonographic measurements in normal pregnancies. Hum Reprod 1996; 11:1771–4.

23. Yapar EG, Ekici E, Gokmen O. First trimester fetal heart rate measurements by transvaginal ultrasound combined with pulsed Doppler: an evaluation of 1331 cases. Eur J Obstet Gynecol Reprod Biol 1995; 60:133–7.

24. Monteagudo A, Timor-Tritsch IE. First trimester anatomy scan: pushing the limits. What can we see now? Curr Opin Obstet Gynecol 2003; 15:131–41.

25. Blaas HG, Eik-Nes SH, Kiserud T, Hellevik LR. Early development of the hindbrain: a longitudinal study from 7 to 12 weeks gestation. Ultrasound Obstet Gynecol 1995; 5:148–9.

26. Hadlock FP, Shah YP, Kanon DJ, Lindsey JV. Fetal crown–rump length: reevaluation of relation to menstrual age (5–18 weeks) with high resolution real time US. Radiology 1992; 182:501–5.

27. Blaas HG, Eik-Nes SH, Kiserud T, Hellevik LR. Early development of the abdominal wall, stomach and heart from 7–12 weeks gestation: a longitudinal ultrasound study. Ultrasound Obstet Gynecol 1995; 6:240–9.

28. Jauniaux E, Gulbis B. Fluid compartments of the embryonic environment. Hum Reprod Update 2000; 6:268–78.

29. Green JJ, Hobbins JC. Abdominal ultrasound examination of the first trimester fetus. Am J Obstet Gynecol 1988; 159:165–75.

30. Gembruch U, Shi C, Smrcek JM. Biometry of the fetal heart between 10 and 17 weeks of gestation. Fetal Diagn Ther 2000; 15:20–31.

31. Haak MC, Twisk JW, Van Vugt JM. How successful is fetal echocardiographic examination in the first trimester of pregnancy? Ultrasound Obstet Gynecol 2002; 20:9–13.

32. Johnson SP, Sebire NJ, Snijders RJM, Tunkel S, Nicolaides KH. Ultrasound screening for anencephaly at 10–14 weeks gestation. Ultrasound Obstet Gynecol 1997; 9:14–16.

33. Achiron R, Tadmor O. Screening for fetal anomalies during the first trimester of pregnancy: transvaginal versus transabdominal sonography. Ultrasound Obstet Gynecol 1991; 1:186–91.

34. Cullen MT, Green J, Whetham J, et al. Transvaginal ultrasonographic detection of congenital anomalies in the first trimester. Am J Obstet Gynecol 1990; 163:466–76.

35. Braithwaite JM, Armstrong MA, Economides DL. Assessment of fetal anatomy at 12 to 13 weeks of gestation by transbdominal and transvaginal sonography. Br J Obstet Gynaecol 1996; 103:83–5.

36. Timor-Tritsch IE, Bashiri A, Monteagudo A, Arslan AA. Qualified and trained sonographers in the US can perform early fetal anatomy scans between 11 and 14 weeks. Am J Obstet Gynecol 2004; 191:1247–52.

37. Economides DL, Whitlow BJ, Kadir R, Lazanakis M, Verdin SM. First trimester sonographic detection of chromosomal abnormalities in an unselected population. Br J Obstet Gynaecol 1998; 105:58–62.

38. Weisz B, Pajkrt E, Jauniaux E. Early detection of fetal structural abnormalities. RBM Online 2005; 10:541–53.

3

Bleeding and pain in early pregnancy: what are the likely problems?

George Condous

Introduction • Transvaginal versus transabdominal approach • Timing of the first transvaginal ultrasound • Clinical symptoms and risk factors for ectopic pregnancy • Incidence and mortality of ectopic pregnancy • Threatened miscarriage • Complete miscarriage • Ovarian cysts in early pregnancy • Other causes of bleeding and pain in early pregnancy • Conclusions • Practical points

INTRODUCTION

For years, medical students have been taught that all pregnant women who present with lower abdominal pain and/or vaginal bleeding in the first trimester have an ectopic pregnancy until proven otherwise. Nothing has changed. Not only is the early diagnosis of ectopic pregnancy in clinically stable women with transvaginal ultrasonography (TVS) potentially life-saving, it may also decrease the number of operative procedures such as diagnostic laparoscopy and dilatation and curettage.[1] The earlier an unruptured ectopic pregnancy is diagnosed, the greater are the treatment options. These not only include conservative management with methotrexate,[2] but also an expectant 'wait and see' approach.[3]

All women of reproductive age with lower abdominal pain, abnormal vaginal bleeding or even gastrointestinal symptoms who present to general practitioners or emergency departments should have a urinary pregnancy test (positive at serum human chorionic gonadotrophin (hCG) levels ≥25 IU/L). The burden of responsibility rests on the shoulders of clinicians – not considering an ectopic pregnancy was a common theme in the most recent Confidential Enquiries into Maternal Deaths (CEMD) in the United Kingdom (UK). In the CEMD, 11 out of

15 direct deaths in the first trimester were due to ectopic pregnancy.[4]

TRANSVAGINAL VERSUS TRANSABDOMINAL APPROACH

This should no longer be a debate. If the urinary pregnancy test is positive, TVS should be performed, preferably in a dedicated Early Pregnancy Unit (EPU) by an ultrasonographer or gynaecologist trained in the management of early pregnancy complications. Not only does TVS confirm viability and gestation, but most importantly it confirms the location of the pregnancy.[5,6] In a recent study of 6621 consecutive women, 91.2% had their pregnancy location confirmed at the initial TVS.[7] In approximately 10% of women, there is no clear evidence of an intrauterine pregnancy, ectopic pregnancy or retained products of conception at the initial scan and these women are classified as pregnancies of unknown location (PUL). The management of these women is discussed in detail in Chapter 7.[8,9]

TVS, when used as a single test, can positively identify an ectopic pregnancy where present (see Figures 3.1 and 3.2). Although in the past few clinicians would use ultrasound

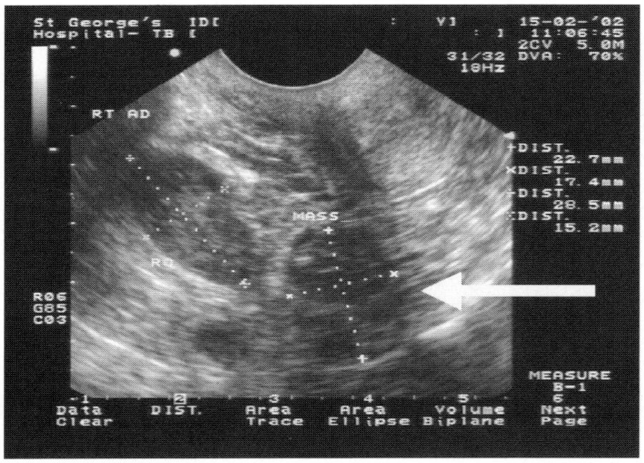

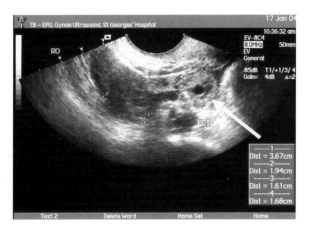

Figure 3.1 Tubal ectopic pregnancy; solid arrow highlights an inhomogeneous mass or 'blob sign' on transvaginal scan. (Reproduced from Kirk et al. Ultrasound Obstet Gynecol 2005; in press.)

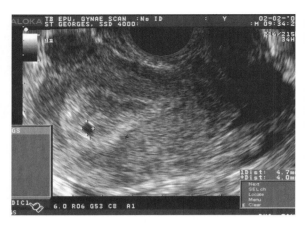

Figure 3.3 Early intrauterine gestational sac; seen as a hyperechoic ring eccentrically placed within the endometrial cavity on transvaginal scan.

Figure 3.2 Tubal ectopic pregnancy; seen as a tubal ring or the bagel sign on transvaginal scan.

control. The so-called 'pseudo sac' is a misnomer and probably represents a fluid collection or debris in the cavity as discussed in the previous chapter. Using high-resolution vaginal probes, it is possible to distinguish an early gestational sac (Figure 3.3) from intracavity fluid, thus making misinterpretation less likely. The standard of care in any EPU can be partly judged by its false-positive and false-negative rates for the diagnosis of ectopic pregnancy. The data to support this view are discussed in greater detail in Chapter 8.

TIMING OF THE FIRST TRANSVAGINAL ULTRASOUND

Some units in the UK do not offer ultrasound scans to women in the first trimester until after 7 weeks' gestation. Such a policy is potentially dangerous as many ectopic pregnancies present before this gestation. In our experience, women with lower abdominal pain and a history of ectopic pregnancy presented at a mean gestation of 20 days.[7]

CLINICAL SYMPTOMS AND RISK FACTORS FOR ECTOPIC PREGNANCY

When evaluating pregnant women in the first trimester, it is very important to take into account the history and symptomatology. The

evidence of an extrauterine pregnancy as the primary way to diagnose ectopic pregnancies, our data suggest that ultrasound is a reliable diagnostic tool.[7] Ectopic pregnancy should not be diagnosed on the basis of an absent intrauterine gestational sac, but rather by the positive visualization of an adnexal mass using two-dimensional grey-scale TVS. If an ectopic pregnancy is present, between 87% and 93% should be identified using TVS prior to surgery.[7–11] Such high detection rates are achievable with adequate training and quality

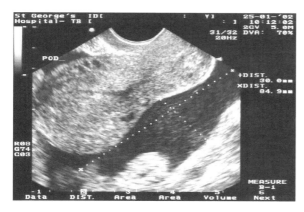

Figure 3.4 Blood in the pouch of Douglas; seen as ground glass fluid on transvaginal scan. (Reproduced from Condous et al. Ultrasound Obstet Gynecol 2003; 2:420–30.)

probability of an ectopic pregnancy is higher in women with clinical symptoms. For example, a woman with a previous ectopic pregnancy who presents with unilateral iliac fossa pain is more likely to have an ectopic pregnancy than an asymptomatic woman in her first pregnancy. Hence the result of an ultrasound scan is influenced by the prior odds.[12] According to a meta-analysis, risk factors for ectopic pregnancy include previous ectopic pregnancy, previous tubal surgery, documented tubal pathology and previous genital infections, including PID, Chlamydia and gonorrhoea.[13] In another study, contraception and the risk of ectopic pregnancy has also been evaluated.[14] Although women becoming pregnant after sterilization or while currently using an intrauterine contraceptive device are at an increased risk of ectopic pregnancy should they become pregnant, neither is a risk factor for ectopic pregnancy.[14]

Pregnant women whose ultrasound in the first trimester demonstrates haemoperitoneum (Figure 3.4) will often, but not always, have abdominal pain. This ultrasound finding is generally thought to be associated with tubal rupture. In fact although the incidence of haemoperitoneum is between 18% and 34%[7,15,16] this does not necessarily mean that tubal rupture has occurred. The majority of ectopic pregnancies with blood in the pouch of Douglas have 'leakage' from the lumen of the fimbrial

end of the fallopian tube. It is very difficult to quantify the volume of haemoperitoneum on an ultrasound scan. However, the presence of blood in Morrison's pouch can be used as a marker for significant haemoperitoneum. In these circumstances clinically one would expect shoulder-tip pain, but this is not always the case. Morrison's pouch is the potential space between Glisson's capsule of the liver and Gerota's fascia surrounding the kidney. Morrison's pouch along with Douglas' pouch are the most sensitive areas for the detection of free intraperitoneal fluid.

INCIDENCE AND MORTALITY OF ECTOPIC PREGNANCY

Whilst the incidence of ectopic pregnancy has progressively increased, the morbidity and associated mortality have substantially decreased. Over 10 000 ectopic pregnancies are diagnosed annually in the UK. The incidence of ectopic pregnancy in the UK is 9.6/1000 pregnancies and the mortality is 4/1000 ectopic pregnancies.[1] The ratio of intra- to extrauterine pregnancies may be as high as 50:1. In tertiary referral EPUs, as many as 3% of women may have an underlying ectopic pregnancy. A total of 95% of ectopic pregnancies are tubal and the majority of these are located in the ampullary region of the fallopian tube. Non-tubal ectopic pregnancies (5%) will be discussed in detail in Chapter 12.

Although spontaneous heterotopic pregnancy is rare (between 1:10 000 and 1:50 000), the incidence is as high as 1% in women following ARTs.[18] In these women, even more care must be taken when inspecting the adnexae using TVS even when an intrauterine sac has been visualized. In our unit, three heterotopic pregnancies have been seen in the last 4 years, one spontaneous and two following ARTs. In the last two cases, although an intrauterine sac was visualized on TVS, these women were admitted with ongoing lower abdominal pain, but were not diagnosed until the time of laparoscopy for declining clinical condition. The management of ectopic pregnancy is discussed in detail in Chapters 9–13.

THREATENED MISCARRIAGE

Women who present in the first trimester with vaginal bleeding with or without lower abdominal pain are given the label of a threatened miscarriage. This is a common first trimester problem occurring in up to one-third of pregnancies.[19] This condition requires an ultrasound scan to establish the viability of the pregnancy. If the uterus contains an embryo-positive cardiac activity, then the woman can be reassured that she has a viable intrauterine pregnancy. If the crown–rump length (CRL) is at least 6 mm and there is no fetal cardiac activity or if the crown rump length is >6 mm with no change at the time of a repeat scan 7 days later, this was formally classified as a missed miscarriage or more recently as 'early fetal demise'.[20] Care must be taken when making this diagnosis, as approximately one-third of embryos with a CRL of less than 5 mm have no demonstrable cardiac activity; under such circumstances a repeat scan should be performed in 7 days.[21] If the uterus contains an empty gestational sac of >20 mm on TVS, this was previously described as an anembryonic pregnancy or blighted ovum. More recent nomenclature has termed this as 'early embryonic demise'. An interval scan in 7 days is recommended if there is any doubt.[20]

Subchorionic haematomas are common and seen in up to 18% of women with a threatened miscarriage.[21] They are insignificant sonographic findings and there is no association between the rate of premature delivery and haematoma size.[22] The confirmation of fetal cardiac activity in a threatened miscarriage confers an excellent prognosis.[23] The management of miscarriage is covered in depth in Chapters 5 and 6.

COMPLETE MISCARRIAGE

This should not be based on an ultrasound diagnosis. Women who present with heavy vaginal bleeding with clots and undergo an ultrasound scan which suggests a complete miscarriage (i.e. an empty uterus with an endometrial thickness less than 15 mm), should be followed up with serum hCG levels until the diagnosis is established.[24] We have described

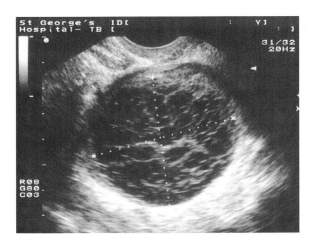

Figure 3.5 Haemorrhagic corpus luteum; classic internal 'spider web'-like appearance on transvaginal scan.

how 5.9% of women with an apparent complete miscarriage have an underlying ectopic pregnancy. A diagnosis of complete miscarriage based on history and scan findings alone is unreliable. Our data highlight the need to classify these cases as PULs. The term 'complete miscarriage' should no longer be used in the context of an ultrasound scan report. All such women should be managed under the umbrella term of PUL until serum hCG levels demonstrate the outcome of the pregnancy. In the most recent CEMD, one potentially avoidable death was in a woman in whom an ultrasonically empty uterus was interpreted as showing a complete miscarriage. According to the CEMD, 'quantitative hCG testing would certainly have established the correct diagnosis'.[4]

OVARIAN CYSTS IN EARLY PREGNANCY

Women who present with lower abdominal pain or unilateral iliac fossa pain need to have a TVS in order to exclude an ectopic pregnancy. In the situation where an intrauterine pregnancy is confirmed, an ovarian cyst may be the cause of the abdominal pain. In a recent study in our unit, we reported that the prevalence of ovarian cysts of ≥25 mm in the first-trimester population studied was 5.4%; the vast majority of these were incidental findings.[25] The

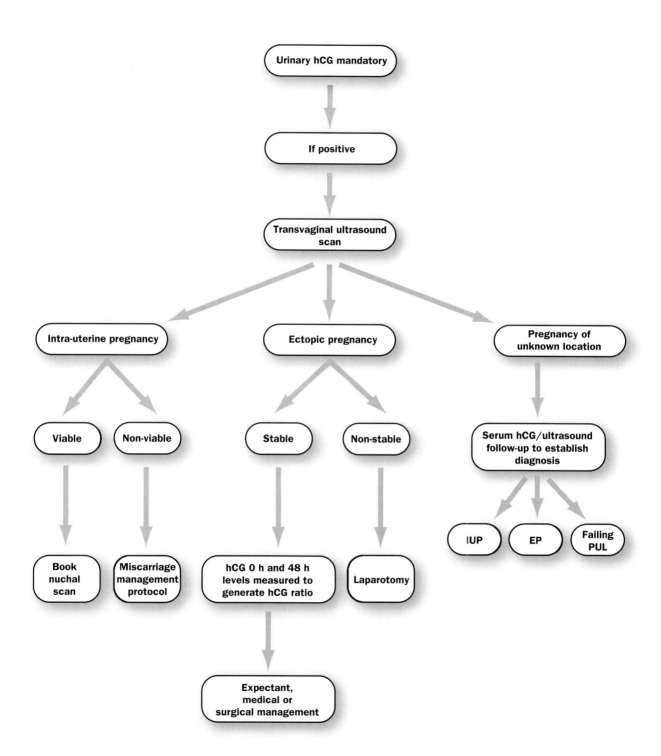

Figure 3.6 Flow diagram to illustrate a suggested management plan for women who present with lower abdominal pain with or without vaginal bleeding in the first trimester.

vast majority of these ovarian cysts resolved spontaneously and expectant management was found to be safe.

Most ovarian cysts in early pregnancy are corpora lutea (Figure 3.5) and these can cause abdominal pain if they undergo haemorrhage, rupture or torsion. The first two complications tend to be self-limiting; however the latter can be catastrophic resulting in ovarian infarction and loss of the ovary if not diagnosed promptly. The diagnosis of ovarian torsion is a clinical one and ultrasound is not always decisive. The management and characterization of ovarian cysts in early pregnancy is covered in Chapter 15. Interestingly, in early pregnancy, localizing the corpus luteum can be a useful guide when looking for an ectopic pregnancy with TVS. It will be on the ipsilateral side in 70–85% of cases.[7,26,27]

OTHER CAUSES OF BLEEDING AND PAIN IN EARLY PREGNANCY

Other causes of abdominal pain in early pregnancy may or may not be related to the pregnancy. Urinary tract infection and surgical causes of abdominal pain such as appendicitis,

cholecystitis, etc. must be considered where appropriate.

Other causes of vaginal bleeding in early pregnancy including molar pregnancy (gestational trophoblastic disease) will not be discussed in this chapter.

One must always consider lower genital tract causes of vaginal bleeding such as cervical polyps, cervical ectropion and in extremely rare cases cervical carcinoma, which has a reported incidence of 1 in 2000 pregnancies.[28]

CONCLUSIONS

All pregnant women who present with lower abdominal pain and/or vaginal bleeding in the first trimester should undergo transvaginal ultrasonography. This confirms viability and gestation but most importantly localizes the pregnancy, enabling appropriate management of women with early pregnancy complications. It is important to remember that the ultrasound findings should not be taken in isolation and the overall clinical scenario should always be considered. The management of the conditions touched on briefly here are discussed in detail in forthcoming chapters.

PRACTICAL POINTS

1. All pregnant women who present with lower abdominal pain and/or vaginal bleeding in the first trimester have an ectopic pregnancy until proven otherwise.

2. All women of reproductive age with lower abdominal pain, abnormal vaginal bleeding or even gastrointestinal symptoms who present to general practitioners or accident and emergency departments should have a urinary pregnancy test (positive at serum hCG levels ≤25 IU/L).

3. Transvaginal ultrasonography and not transabdominal should be the primary imaging modality in the assessment of women in the first trimester.

4. Transvaginal ultrasonography not only confirms viability and gestation of an early pregnancy, but most importantly confirms the location of the pregnancy.

5. Transvaginal ultrasonography when used as a single test can positively identify an ectopic pregnancy where present.

6. The timing of the first ultrasound scan should not be determined by the gestation of the pregnancy.

7. Risk factors for ectopic pregnancy include previous ectopic pregnancy, previous tubal surgery, documented tubal pathology and previous genital infections, including PID, *Chlamydia* and gonorrhoea.

8. Although women becoming pregnant after sterilization or while currently using an intrauterine contraceptive device are at an increased risk of ectopic pregnancy, neither is a risk factor for ectopic pregnancy.

9. The incidence of ectopic pregnancy in the United Kingdom is 9.6/1000 pregnancies and the mortality is 4/1000 ectopic pregnancies.
10. Spontaneous heterotopic pregnancy is rare (between 1:10 000 and 1:50 000), but the incidence is as high as 1% in women following ARTs.
11. Subchorionic haematomas are common and seen in up to 18% of women with a threatened miscarriage.
12. Subchorionic haematomas are insignificant sonographic findings and there is no association between the rate of premature delivery and haematoma size.
13. 'Complete miscarriage' should no longer be used and all such women should be managed under the umbrella term of PUL.
14. The amount of bleeding does not always indicate the likely problem. Heavy bleeding does not always indicate a miscarriage.

REFERENCES

1. Atri M, Valenti DA, Bret PM, et al. Effect of transvaginal sonography on the use of invasive procedures for evaluating patients with a clinical diagnosis of ectopic pregnancy. J Clin Ultrasound 2003; 31:1–8.
2. Hajenius PJ, Engelsbel S, Mol BW, et al. Randomised trial of systemic methotrexate versus laparoscopic salpingostomy. Lancet 1997; 350:774–9.
3. Korhonen J, Stenman UH, Ylostalo P. Serum human chorionic gonadotropin dynamics during spontaneous resolution of ectopic pregnancy. Fertil Steril 1994; 61:632–6.
4. Lewis G, Drife J, editors. Why Mothers Die, Triennial Report 2000–2002. The Sixth Report of the Confidential Enquiries into Maternal Deaths in the United Kingdom. RCOG Press, 2004.
5. Condous G, Okaro E, Bourne T. The conservative management of early pregnancy complications: a review of the literature. Ultrasound Obstet Gynecol 2003; 22:420–30.
6. Condous G. The management of early pregnancy complications. Best Pract Res Clin Obstet Gynaecol 2004; 18:37–57.
7. Condous G, Okaro E, Khalid A, Lu C, Van Huffel S, Bourne T. The accuracy of transvaginal ultrasonography for the diagnosis of ectopic pregnancy prior to surgery. Hum Reprod 2005; 20:1404–9.
8. Banerjee S, Aslam N, Woelfer B, et al. Expectant management of early pregnancies of unknown location: a prospective evaluation of methods to predict spontaneous resolution of pregnancy. Br J Obstet Gynaecol 2001; 108:158–63.
9. Condous G, Lu C, Van Huffel S, Timmerman D, Bourne T. Human chorionic gonadotrophin and progesterone levels for the investigation of pregnancies of unknown location. Int J Gynecol Obstet 2004; 86:351–7.
10. Shalev E, Yarom I, Bustan M, et al. Transvaginal sonography as the ultimate diagnostic tool for the management of ectopic pregnancy: experience with 840 cases. Fert Steril 1998; 69:62–5.
11. Cacciatore B, Stenman UH, Ylostalo P. Diagnosis of ectopic pregnancy by vaginal ultrasonography in combination with a discriminatory serum hCG level of 1000 IU/L (IRP). Br J Obstet Gynaecol 1990; 97:904–8.
12. Hall GH. The clinical application of Bayes' theorem. Lancet 1967; 9:555–7.
13. Ankum WM, Mol BW, Van der Veen F, et al. Risk factors for ectopic pregnancy: a meta-analysis. Fertil Steril 1997; 65:1093–9.
14. Mol BW, Ankum WM, Bossuyt PM, et al. Contraception and the risk of ectopic pregnancy. Contraception 1995; 52:337–41.
15. DiMarchi JM, Kosasa TS, Hale RW. What is the significance of the human chorionic gonadotropin value in ectopic pregnancy? Obstet Gynecol 1989; 74:851–5.
16. Saxon D, Falcone T, Mascha EJ, et al. A study of ruptured tubal ectopic pregnancy. Obstet Gynecol 1997; 90:46–9.
17. Kirk E, Condous G, Bourne T. Ectopic pregnancy deaths: what should we be doing? Hosp Medicine 2004; 65:657–60
18. Ludwig M, Kaisi M, Bauer O, et al. Heterotopic pregnancy in a spontaneous cycle: do not forget about it! Eur J Obstet Gynecol Reprod Biol 1999; 87:91–3.
19. Sieroszewski P, Suzin J, Bernaschek G, et al. Evaluation of first trimester pregnancy in cases of threatened abortion by means of doppler sonography. Ultraschall 2001; 22:208–12.

20. Luise C, Jermy K, Collins WP, et al. Outcome of expectant management of spontaneous first trimester miscarriage: observational study. BMJ 2002; 324:873–5.

21. Levi CS, Lyons EA, Zheng XH, et al. Endovaginal Ultrasound: demonstration of cardiac activity in embryos less than 5.0 mm in crown–rump length. Radiology 1990; 176:71–4.

22. Pedersen JF, Mantoni M. Prevalence and significance of subchorionic hemorrhage in threatened abortion: a sonographic study. Am J Roentgenol 1990; 154: 535–7.

23. Mantoni M. Ultrasound signs in threatened abortion and their prognostic significance. Obstet Gynecol 1985; 65:471–5.

24. Condous G, Okaro E, Khalid A, Bourne T. Do we need to follow up complete miscarriages with serum human chorionic gonadotrophin levels? Br J Obstet Gynaecol 2005; 112:827–9.

25. Condous G, Khalid A, Okaro E, Bourne T. Should we be examining the ovaries in pregnancy? The natural history of adnexal pathology detected at first trimester ultrasonography. Ultrasound Obstet Gynecol 2004; 24:62–6.

26. Walters MD, Eddy C, Pauerstein CJ. The contralateral corpus luteum and tubal pregnancy. Obstet Gynecol 1987; 70: 823–6.

27. Jurkovic D, Bourne TH, Jauniaux E, et al. Transvaginal color Doppler study of blood flow in ectopic pregnancies. Fertil Steril 1992; 57: 68–73.

28. Nevin J, Soefers R, Dahaeck K, et al. Cervical carcinoma associated with pregnancy. Obstet Gynecol Surv 1995; 50:228.

4

The diagnosis of miscarriage

Steven R Goldstein

Introduction • Definitions • Risk factors and aetiology for pregnancy failure • Embryonic losses • Normal ultrasonographic milestones in early pregnancy • When are serial hCG determinations appropriate? • Conclusions • Practical points

INTRODUCTION

Miscarriage is a term often used interchangeably with complete miscarriage by the lay public and even medical professionals. A better term for the healthcare professional involved in an Early Pregnancy Unit is 'early pregnancy failure'. Any chapter entitled 'The diagnosis of miscarriage' has to begin with some housekeeping by defining varying terms that are often confused. The definitions used in clinical practice are unsatisfactory and need to be rationalized. Some reflect the clinical presentation and others the findings on ultrasonography. Some miscarriages will be obvious because of the presence of pregnancy products in the cervix or vagina. In reality, prior to an ultrasound scan, in most cases the problem can only be classified as 'bleeding and pain in early pregnancy'. An accurate diagnosis will only be possible in most cases after an ultrasound scan and in some following the measurement of serial levels of serum hCG. However for the sake of completeness the following are commonly used definitions.

DEFINITIONS

Threatened miscarriage: Clinically if women present in the first trimester with vaginal bleeding with or without lower abdominal pain (cervical os is closed) they are labelled as a 'threatened miscarriage'. This very common problem requires an ultrasound scan to establish the viability of the pregnancy.

Complete miscarriage: Clinically the products of conception have totally passed; the cervix is likely to be closed on examination; bleeding and cramping should have diminished. A transvaginal ultrasound scan (TVS) demonstrates a thin endometrial thickness (often defined as <15 mm). These women should be treated as a pregnancy of unknown location (PUL) if they have not had a previous scan to confirm the location. Follow-up serum human chorionic gonadotrophin (hCG) levels should be performed to confirm the outcome of pregnancy failure.

Incomplete miscarriage: Clinically partial passage of the products of conception, bleeding and cramping is variable; characterized by an open cervical os on physical examination. Products of conception may be seen in the cervical os or vagina. TVS demonstrates heterogeneous material within the endometrial cavity. In most cases the condition does not require dilatation and curettage (D&C) and if managed expectantly will have 90% successful resolution.

Early embryonic demise (previously termed an anembryonic pregnancy or blighted ovum): If the uterus contains an empty gestational sac of >20 mm on TVS, this almost certainly represents early embryonic demise, however an interval scan in 7 days or for the findings to be checked by a second operator is recommended if there is any doubt.

Early fetal demise (previously termed missed miscarriage): This is a failed pregnancy of up to 12 weeks; definitively non-viable but not yet passed. If the CRL is at least 6 mm and there is no fetal cardiac activity or if the crown–rump length is > 6 mm with no change at the time of a repeat scan 7 days later, this is classified as early fetal demise. This is sometimes treated expectantly, medically or electively removed by D&C. (This often depends on gestational age, the size of pregnancy as well as the availability of resources and the woman's preference.)

RISK FACTORS AND AETIOLOGY FOR PREGNANCY FAILURE

Risk factors include advancing maternal age, previous failed pregnancy, smoking, moderate to heavy alcohol use, cocaine, NSAIDs/aspirin (by interference with prostaglandins), fever, caffeine (dose related, questionably secondary to cytochrome P450 enzyme activation) and low folate.

The aetiology of pregnancy failure is complicated and could be the subject of an entire chapter. Suffice it to say that it can be associated with chromosomal abnormalities. Pregnancies associated with trisomy 21, 18 and 13 are the most likely to survive. All other trisomies end in early pregnancy failure. Congenital anomalies are also a source of pregnancy failure. Maternal endocrinopathies, especially diabetes, and haemoglobin A1C levels at conception correlate with risk of pregnancy failure. Other related conditions include uterine abnormalities (adhesions, septae and submucous fibroids). Acute or chronic maternal illness and/or infection can result in early pregnancy failure. Thrombophilia as well as auto-immune disorders are controversial as to their role, if any, in early pregnancy failure and recurrent miscarriage in particular.

Our modern understanding of early pregnancy and its failure results from firstly the ability to detect minute levels of serum hCG, secondly lessons learned from the assisted reproductive technologies and finally from the improved resolution available using TVS.

Serum hCG is produced by trophoblastic tissue. It is detectable 8 days post conception.

Erroneously it is still referred to by some as a 'beta subunit' or simply 'beta' to distinguish it from the alpha subunit shared with TSH and other molecules. Most current tests however measure the intact hCG molecule. Over-the-counter home pregnancy tests will turn positive at or around the time of the missed menses at a level of 25 IU/L. Serum hCG normally rises by a minimum of 66% every 48 hours although it often doubles in that period of time. A total of 15–20% of ectopic pregnancies will follow a normal doubling time of hCG. These are the ones that will usually end up with an embryo and/or heart beat in an extrauterine location. Most normal early pregnancies are seen on TVS once the serum hCG level is >1000 IU/L. Thus there may be a variable but lengthy period of time from when a woman can diagnose a pregnancy event with a home pregnancy test and when one will first be able to visualize it.

TVS provides a degree of image magnification that is as if we were performing ultrasonography through a low power microscope ('sonomicroscopy'). Prior to the vaginal probe, ultrasonography was a tool mainly of the obstetrician. Early equipment had barely enough resolution for limited functions such as placental localization, establishing fetal lie, and to perform measurements of gestational age based on parameters such as the biparietal diameter and crown–rump length.

Several decades of conventional wisdom taught us that '25% of all pregnancies will experience bleeding in the first trimester and of those half will miscarry'. Such women were often told to go home, put their feet up and that they had a 50/50 chance of the pregnancy continuing. Although these statistics are very close to accurate, modern practice allows us to tell such women much more. The outcome, however, will usually remain the same.

A biochemical pregnancy has been defined as a pregnancy detected by assays of serum hCG but one that has failed before it can be clinically recognized (as bleeding then occurs at or around the time of the expected menses). Wilcox et al.[1] studied 221 women attempting to conceive by measuring daily hCG levels by radioimmunoassay. Twenty-two per cent of pregnancies detected by assay were lost prior to clinical recognition. However, of these, 35% became clinically pregnant the next cycle, 65% clinically pregnant by the third cycle and 83% by the sixth cycle. Such a chemical pregnancy is an excellent prognostic sign indicating that the woman is ovulatory, has tubal patency (at least on one side), has a fertile partner and is herself capable of capacitating her partner's semen.

Now that women have the ability to clinically recognize their own pregnancies by the time of their missed menses, a more appropriate definition of chemical pregnancy would be one in which loss occurs prior to the onset of the embryonic period.

EMBRYONIC LOSSES

The embryonic period is a 5-week window from 21 days' post conception (5 weeks from the last menstrual period (LMP)) when the endothelial heart tube folds on itself and begins to beat. It is a time of organogenesis and thus concerns about teratogens are real. It concludes at 70 days LMP (10 weeks) when organ system development is complete and the embryo now becomes a fetus (the word itself from the Latin meaning 'having a human-like appearance').

Numerous authors have looked at the role of chromosomal abnormalities in these embryonic losses. One study[2] looked at 144 spontaneous miscarriages by obtaining direct preparations of chorionic villi. Seventy per cent had abnormal chromosomes of which 64% were autosomal trisomies, 9% polyploidy, 7% monosomy X and 6% structural rearrangements.

Errors of gonadogenesis during meiosis will result in autosomal trisomies. Errors of fertilization can result in triploidy from dispermy. Errors of the first division of the zygote result in tetraploidy or mosaicism. None of these would be expected to be a repetitive event except in the very rare instances of balanced translocations or inversions in one parent.

The other 30% of non-chromosomal early pregnancy failures will include uterine abnormalities, infectious agents (T strain mycoplasmas), maternal alcohol, maternal smoking, molecular genetic abnormalities with normal karyotypes, possibly autoimmune factors, and questionably luteal phase defects.

Some authors[3] have suggested that karyotyping chorionic villi obtained at the time of curettage for failed pregnancies prior to spontaneous passage can serve a valuable clinical role. The presence of abnormal chromosomes gives the parents a definitive diagnosis as to why the pregnancy failed and may obviate the need for further investigation. Karyotyping a failed pregnancy that produces normal chromosomes can potentially result in the search for various other causes without the couple first having to go through a subsequent failed pregnancy.

The natural history of pregnancy failure in the general population has long been of interest to clinicians. Simpson et al.[4] found that most losses although not clinically encountered until after 8 weeks actually occur prior to 8 weeks. Spontaneous passage of products of conception actually occurs 1–4 weeks after an embryo loses its viability. It is very important that women understand that rarely is physical activity on the day of spontaneous passage the cause of pregnancy loss. Such an event means that the pregnancy had usually been non-viable for more than 1 week.

Another study[5] looked at 232 women with no bleeding prior to the first visit. All women had a TVS at the initial visit and at all subsequent visits up to 12 weeks. The latest anatomical landmark visualized using ultrasonography was recorded. There were 200 births, 27 embryonic losses and five fetal losses. These authors looked at loss rates subsequently in the embryonic period based on the anatomical landmark achieved. Thus, if a pregnancy developed to the stage of visualizing a gestational sac, there was still a subsequent loss rate in the embryonic period of 11.5%. If the pregnancy developed a yolk sac visible on ultrasound, the subsequent loss rate in the embryonic period was 8.5%. The development of an embryo to over 5 mm was associated with a 7.2% loss rate in the embryonic period. Embryos of more than 1 cm had a subsequent loss in the embryonic period of 0.5%. The authors did report a 2.4% loss in the fetal period due to factors such as an incompetent cervix, severe maternal infection and abnormalities of placentation. This is in contrast with the 70% of embryonic losses that are thought to be chromosomal.

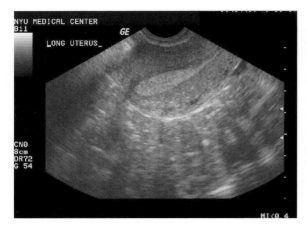

Figure 4.1 Longitudinal axis view of the uterus on transvaginal ultrasonography of a woman with uncertain dates. An over-the-counter home pregnancy test was positive and the woman had a 2-day history of vaginal staining. The cervical os was closed. This endometrial echo is homogeneous and thick, and is compatible with but not diagnostic of a normal early ongoing pregnancy. The quantitative hCG level was 425 mIU/ml. Staining persisted and a follow-up scan in 96 hours revealed a definitive intrauterine gestational sac.

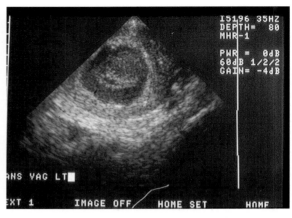

Figure 4.2 Transvaginal pelvic ultrasound scan on a woman with a positive home pregnancy test and vaginal bleeding. The endometrial appearance here, suggestive of blood debris and clot, is compatible with a failed intrauterine pregnancy or possibly ectopic pregnancy. This appearance however cannot support the existence of an early ongoing intrauterine pregnancy.

Thus it becomes readily apparent that the key to successful use of early pregnancy ultrasound depends on knowing what early pregnancy looks like using ultrasonography and why (covered in Chapter 3) and being able to differentiate between pregnancies with acceptable growth and continued wellbeing and those pregnancies that are absolutely destined to fail.

NORMAL ULTRASONOGRAPHIC MILESTONES IN EARLY PREGNANCY

The threshold level is the earliest that a structure can be visualized using TVS (e.g. gestational sac, yolk sac, cardiac activity). The discriminatory level is the point at which a structure must be visualized if it is normal.

When should you see a gestational sac?

Usually by 5 weeks LMP (3 weeks post conception) a gestational sac will be visualized. However, virtually all clinicians know that menstrual dating is notoriously unreliable.

Therefore the concept of a discriminatory level of hCG was developed. The discriminatory level of hCG was originally described in 1981.[6] The initial report was with transabdominal ultrasound and equalled 6500 IU/L. This was updated in 1985 by Nyberg et al.[7] to 3600 IU/L. Transvaginal ultrasonography led to the level being reduced to 1000 IU/L.[8] Clearly this will depend on the type and frequency of the equipment used, its degree of magnification, as well as the presence of coexisting fibroids. Furthermore it can be affected by extreme maternal obesity, the uterus being in a poor scanning position (e.g. axial) and in the presence of a multiple pregnancy. The endometrium, while lacking a gestational sac should at least have an appearance compatible with an early normal pregnancy, that is lush, homogeneous and decidualized/secretory in appearance (see Figures 4.1, 4.2 and 4.3). Details of the management when a pregnancy sac cannot be seen in the uterus in the presence of a positive pregnancy test are outside the scope of this chapter (see Chapter 7).

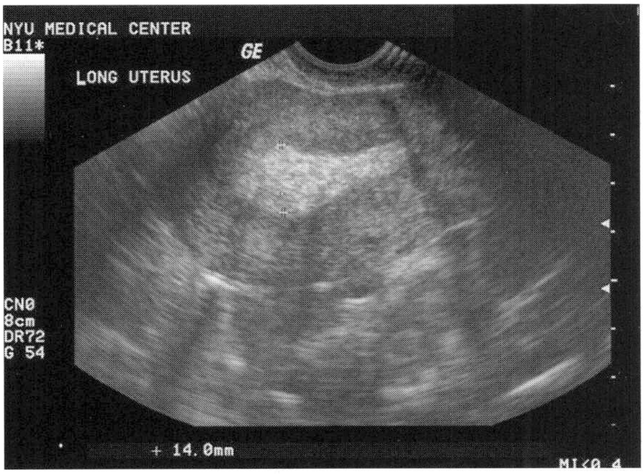

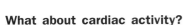

Figure 4.3 Longitudinal axis transvaginal ultrasound view of a woman whose last period was 5^{+6} weeks before but with a history of markedly irregular cycles. The woman had a 2-day history of vaginal spotting and a closed cervical os on physical examination. The home pregnancy test was positive. This appearance of the endometrial echo is at least compatible with an early ongoing intrauterine pregnancy that may just be below the level of the discriminatory zone. A report of 'no gestational sac seen' is inadequate in such cases. It is essential that the findings seem at least be compatible with an ongoing potentially viable intrauterine pregnancy.

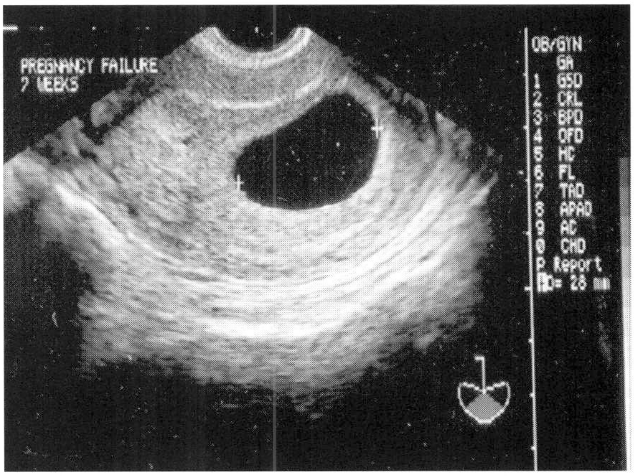

Figure 4.4 Intrauterine gestational sac at 7 weeks. The mean gestation sac diameter was 28 mm. The failure to visualise a normal yolk sac is diagnostic of a definitively failed intrauterine gestation. A follow-up ultrasound scan or serial determination of hCG levels in such a case is unnecessary and inappropriate.

When should you see a yolk sac?

The discriminatory level for a yolk sac with transabdominal ultrasound was a mean gestation sac diameter (MSD) of 20 mm.[9] Early TVS described a discriminatory level for the yolk sac of 8 mm.[10] More recently Rowling et al.[11] found that with 5 MHz transducers the yolk sac is definitively seen by a MSD of 13 mm but with newer 5–9 MHz transducers a yolk sac was definitively seen by the time the MSD was 5 mm. The presence of a larger sac with no evidence of yolk sac formation contained within it is a definitive sign of a non-viable pregnancy (Figure 4.4) In addition an abnormal or hydropic yolk sac is a non-specific sign or 'soft marker' of early pregnancy failure (Figures 4.5 and 4.6).

What about cardiac activity?

The endothelial heart tube folds on itself and begins to beat 21 days post conception. Thus any pregnancy whose outcome is ultimately normal has cardiac activity present in the early

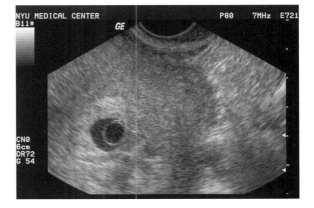

Figure 4.5 A highly magnified view of a gestational sac in a woman at 6^{+4} weeks by her LMP. This scan shows a small sac with a large hydropic (8.5 mm) yolk sac. This picture is compatible with intrauterine pregnancy failure.

embryo prior to our ability to image it. The question is therefore not how early we can see cardiac activity (the threshold level) but at what point if cardiac activity is not seen with TVS is

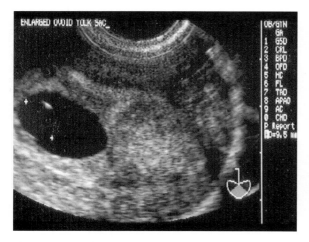

Figure 4.6 A transvaginal scan of a highly magnified gestation sac contained within a decidualized endometrial echo. The yolk sac is hydropic and irregular in shape and measures 9.5 mm (calipers). This picture is typical of intrauterine pregnancy failure.

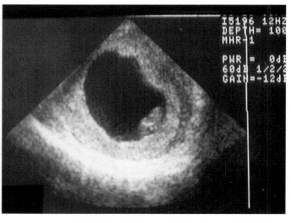

Figure 4.7 A transvaginal scan at 58 days' gestation. A routine scan 9 days previously had revealed an embryo of 7 mm with obvious cardiac activity. She had a 1-day history of vaginal spotting. This scan depicts a 5 mm amorphous embryonic structure without cardiac activity. In previous years with transabdominal ultrasound such a sac appeared 'empty' and was often called an 'anembryonic pregnancy'. More appropriate nomenclature is 'embryonic demise with resorption'.

a pregnancy definitively non viable (the discriminatory level). Levi et al.[12] found that all normal outcomes had cardiac activity by an embryonic size of 4 mm or more. Brown et al.[13] reported one case of a 4 mm embryo in which cardiac activity could not be located but ultimately proved to be normal. Another study[14] found that all cardiac activity ultimately present was seen by an embryonic size of 4 mm or greater (Figure 4.7). The ability to see cardiac activity using ultrasonography will have the same constraints as for visualizing a gestational sac. Although literature exists on the relationship between heart rate and prognosis the reader is cautioned about using such information when counselling women. In a study of 40 women of less than 8 weeks' gestation, when the embryonic heart rate was less than 90 beats per minute (bpm) there was an 80% loss rate, whereas for heart rates between 70 and 79 bpm the loss rate was 91%.[15]

If we ask the rhetorical question: how do we encounter early pregnancies that are failed or 'potentially' failed? The answers would be when we see women who are pregnant with

any pain, bleeding or even staining. All such women require evaluation with TVS. In addition occasionally we encounter women before any bleeding who have definitive ultrasonographic evidence of a failed pregnancy. The criteria for a failed pregnancy (often requiring serial examination) are:

- The failure to image a yolk sac within a gestational sac by the time the gestational sac has reached a mean sac diameter of 5–13 mm (depending on transducer frequency), or an embryo of greater than or equal to 4 mm without cardiac activity.
- The failure of the gestation sac or embryo to grow at the expected rate (1 mm/day).
- The loss of cardiac activity previously documented as being present.

Failure of serum hCG levels to rise at the expected rate are usually diagnostic of an abnormal pregnancy although its location may be uncertain. There are other less specific or 'soft' markers of early pregnancy loss. A yolk sac of greater than 6 mm with or without abnormal

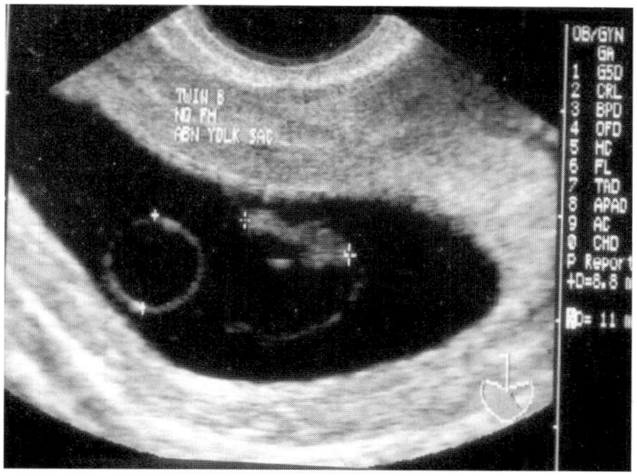

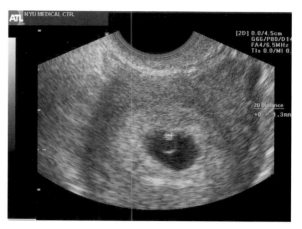

Figure 4.8 A transvaginal scan of a twin pregnancy. An 11 mm embryo without cardiac activity can be seen. Notice the hydropic yolk sac adjacent, measuring 8.0 mm (calipers). This is another example of intrauterine pregnancy failure.

Figure 4.9 This patient was 6^{+1} weeks by her LMP with a 1-day history of vaginal bleeding and a closed cervical os. Ten days previous to this a home pregnancy test was positive. The scan shows a normal-appearing yolk sac with a 1.3 mm embryonic structure identified (calipers). Cardiac activity was not discernible. Follow-up hCG determinations are not appropriate or indicated. A follow-up scan in 1 week revealed an 8 mm embryonic structure with cardiac activity present.

morphology, a mobile gestation sac, disproportionate gestation sac contents or mobile contents are all poor prognostic signs (Figure 4.8).

WHEN ARE SERIAL HCG DETERMINATIONS APPROPRIATE?

Serial hCG determinations are appropriate to exclude ectopic pregnancy in a woman with a serum hCG level below the discriminatory zone in whom there is a concern about the possibility of extrauterine pregnancy. This concept is discussed in detail elsewhere in this book. However once an ectopic pregnancy has been excluded, any assessment of embryonic wellbeing depends on serial ultrasound examinations and not serial hCG determinations. These are unnecessary. Although average serum hCG levels have been published for when various anatomic landmarks are seen sonographically,[10] the 95% confidence intervals of such determinations are so wide as to render them clinically meaningless and potentially dangerous. Once ectopic pregnancy is ruled out the clinician should utilize the fact that the embryo grows

1 mm/day and the gestational sac grows 1 mm/day to assess embryonic wellbeing.

The following two cases illustrate the relevance of follow up using ultrasound to establish the diagnosis and not serial hCG measurements.

CASE REPORT 1

A woman with an uncertain LMP presented with a two-day history of vaginal staining. A home pregnancy test was positive. TVS revealed a gestational sac measuring 4.5 mm MSD. No yolk sac was visualized. The use of serial hCG determination in such a woman is uncalled for and inappropriate. If clinically relevant a follow up scan in 1 week would expect to find an 11–12 mm gestational sac that should contain a yolk sac.

CASE REPORT 2

A woman whose LMP suggested she was between 6 and 7 weeks pregnant, presented with a one-day history of vaginal bleeding (Figure 4.9). Physical examination revealed the cervical os to be closed. A home pregnancy test carried out 10 days previously was positive. TVS revealed an intrauterine gestation sac with a yolk sac and a 1.3 mm embryonic structure identified. Cardiac activity could not be elicited. Follow-up hCG determinations are not indicated. Follow-up TVS in one week revealed an 8 mm embryo with cardiac activity present.

CONCLUSIONS

The modern approach to pregnancy failure requires an understanding of serum hCG changes, ultrasound and the difference between a threshold level and a discriminatory level for features in early pregnancy. Applications of these principles will allow the healthcare professional in the early pregnancy unit to successfully assist women in discriminating between viable ongoing pregnancies and those absolutely destined to fail.

PRACTICAL POINTS

1. The diagnosis of miscarriage should be ultrasound based and not clinical.
2. If there are any doubts about the viability of a pregnancy on TVS, an interval scan should be performed 7 days later.
3. Serum hCG is produced by trophoblastic tissue and is detectable 8 days post conception.
4. Serum hCG normally rises a minimum of 66% every 48 hours (i.e. hCG ratio >1.66) in ongoing intrauterine pregnancies; however this rise can also be seen in 15–20% of ectopic pregnancies.
5. A failure of serum hCG levels to rise at the expected rate is diagnostic of an abnormal pregnancy, although its location may be uncertain..
6. The embryonic period is from 5 weeks gestation and concludes at 70 days gestation.
7. Organogenesis is complete 70 days after the last menstrual period.
8. Up to 70% of spontaneous miscarriages will have an underlying chromosomal abnormality.
9. A gestational sac should be visualized on TVS by 5 weeks gestation.
10. An intrauterine sac should be seen on TVS when the serum level of hCG is above 1000 IU/L.

REFERENCES

1. Wilcox AJ, Weinberg CR, O'Connor JF, et al. Incidence of early loss of pregnancy. N Engl J Med 1988; 319:189–94

2. Ohno M, Maeda T, Matsunobo A. A cytogenetic study of spontaneous abortions with direct analysis of chorionic villi. Obstet Gynecol 1991; 77:394–8.

3. Goldstein SR, Kerenyi T, Scher J, et al. Correlation between karyotype and ultrasound findings in patients with failed early pregnancy. Ultrasound Obstet Gynecol 1996;8:314–317.

4. Simpson JL, Mills JL, Holmes LB, et al. Low fetal loss rates after ultrasound-proved viability in early pregnancy. JAMA 1987; 258:2555–7.

5. Goldstein SR. Early detection of pathologic pregnancy by transvaginal sonography. J Clin Ultrasound 1990; 18:262–73.

6. Kadar N, Devore G, Romero R. Discriminatory hCG zone: its use in the sonographic evaluation for ectopic pregnancy. Obstet Gynecol 1981; 58:156–61.

7. Nyberg DA, Filly RA, Mahony BS, et al. Early gestation: correlation of HCG levels and sonographic identification. Am J Roentgenol 1985; 144: 951–4.

8. Goldstein SR. Early detection of pathologic pregnancy by transvaginal sonography. J Clin Ultrasound 1990; 18:262–73.

9. Nyberg DA, Mack LA, Laing FC, et al. Distinguishing normal from abnormal gestational sac growth in early pregnancy. J Ultrasound Med 1988; 6:23–7.

10. Bree RL, Edwards M, Bohm-Velez M, et al. Transvaginal sonography in the evaluation of normal early pregnancy: correlation with hCG level. Am J Roentgenol 1989; 153:75–9.

11. Rowling SE, Langer JE, Coleman BG, et al. Sonography

during early pregnancy: dependence of threshold and discriminatory values on transvaginal transducer frequency. Am J Roentgenol 1999; 172:983–8.

12. Levi CS, Lyons EA, Zheng XH, et al. Endovaginal US: demonstration of cardiac activity in embryos of less than 5.0 mm in crown–rump length. Radiology 1990; 176:71–4.

13. Brown DL, Emerson DS, Felker RE, et al. Diagnosis of early embryonic demise by endovaginal sonography. J Ultrasound Med 1990; 9:631–6.

14. Goldstein SR. Significance of cardiac activity on endovaginal ultrasound in very early embryos. Obstet Gynecol 1992; 80:670–2

15. Benson CB, Doubilet PM. Slow embryonic heart rate in early first trimester: indicator of poor pregnancy outcome. Radiology 1994; 192:343–4

5

The expectant management of miscarriage

Sven Nielsen and Seth Granberg

Introduction • Diagnostic measures • Treatment of miscarriage • Expectant management of miscarriage • Conclusions • Case report • Practical points

INTRODUCTION

Relatively little was known before the twentieth century about first-trimester miscarriage, probably due to difficulties in diagnosing early pregnancy.

In 1884, Meinl noted selective softening in the lower part of the uterus during vaginal examination in early pregnancy and in 1895 Hegar described signs, symptoms and findings during vaginal examination in early pregnancy in his publication 'Diagnose der frühesten Schwangerschaftsperiode'.[1] Furthermore Aschheim and Zondek, in 1927 and 1928 demonstrated that the urine of pregnant women contained a gonad-stimulating substance which, when injected subcutaneously into female mice, induced follicular maturation.[2] These authors believed that the anterior pituitary produced this gonadotropic substance, but subsequent work by other investigators demonstrated that the placenta was responsible for the production of the hormone and consequently it was given the name human chorionic gonadotrophin (hCG). Immunological pregnancy testing based on antibodies raised against parts of the hCG molecule became available for broad clinical use during the 1960s.[3] Sensitive pregnancy tests made early diagnosis possible and it soon became evident that certain pregnancies were so short-lived that they could only be diagnosed as so-called biochemical pregnancies. This was discussed briefly in the previous chapter.

Based on theoretical calculations, Roberts and Lowe (1975) postulated a 78% failure rate for all human conceptions.[4] Miller and co-workers (1980) observed a 43% pregnancy loss among 152 conceptions in 632 cycles of volunteer women.[5]

In a series where illegal abortions could be excluded, Tietze (1950) calculated that miscarriage occurred in 7% of recognized pregnancies.[6] Clinically recognizable miscarriages today account for about 15% of registered pregnancies.[7-9] Approximately 25% of all women who become pregnant will experience one or more pregnancy losses. The majority of clinically recognizable miscarriages occur before the 13th week (91 days), counted from the last menstrual period.[9-11]

The number of illegal abortions that took place before changes in the legislation concerning early terminations in most parts of the industrialized world is difficult to estimate, since both patient and provider were threatened by prosecution and punishment. The frequency of illegal abortions among women treated in the past under the diagnosis of 'spontaneous' miscarriage has been estimated to be between 10 and 90%.[12-14] Many 'miscarriages' were terminations initiated under poor hygienic conditions by abortionists with only meagre knowledge of the procedure. Illegal terminations were probably the main cause of complications and certainly the cause of both severe bleeding and infection leading occasionally to patient death.[12–14]

The changed legislation concerning termination of early pregnancies has had a profound effect on the frequency of reported miscarriage and the associated complication rate in most Western countries. Unfortunately, criminal abortions are still a reality in many countries where termination of unwanted pregnancies is illegal.[15,16] Illegal abortion is in fact the second most common cause of death in woman between 15 and 40 years of age in many developing countries.[17]

DIAGNOSTIC MEASURES

Clinical

As long ago as 1895, Hegar meticulously described the clinical diagnosis of early pregnancy. Since it is difficult to date a pregnancy before the 8th week by vaginal examination, the length of an early pregnancy is usually estimated from the last menstrual period (LMP).[1,18] Because vaginal bleeding occurs in 25% of normal pregnancies and in the majority of pathological pregnancies, the exact length of a pregnancy complicated by bleeding is often difficult to establish.[19] As Goldstein has previously discussed in Chapter 4, before the era of ultrasound, inevitable miscarriage was considered to be present when pain or bleeding threatened the mother's wellbeing. Incomplete miscarriage when part of the products of conception had passed the cervix, and complete miscarriage when the products of conception had been passed, the uterus was contracted toward normal size and the cervix was closed.[20] As has been discussed in previous chapters, relying on clinical measures alone does not enable the clinician to differentiate between threatening, incomplete and complete miscarriage, ectopic pregnancy, very early normal pregnancy and chorionic malignancies.[19]

Laboratory tests

Accurate immunological pregnancy tests based on detection of urinary hCG at levels from 20 to 50 IU/L are available to the majority of health services today. The advent of sensitive pregnancy tests has helped to improve diagnosis. However, it has also resulted in an increased number of biochemical miscarriages being diagnosed, with a subsequent increase in women classified as recurrent miscarriers.[11]

Measurement of serum levels of hCG, alone or in combination with measurement of progesterone, is useful in daily clinical practice to assess the viability and location of early pregnancies.[19,21,22] Such measurements are of great value in the differentiation between pathological and possible normal pregnancy.[19,22,23] In the case of a known ectopic pregnancy, the combined measurement of hCG and progesterone can be used to identify those ectopics that carry a high risk of complications after conservative treatment.[21,24] These issues will be discussed in more detail in later chapters. The incorporation of new biochemical markers such as the inhibins and insulin growth factor binding proteins into diagnostic models could probably help to select women for different treatment modalities.[25]

Ultrasonography

Wild and Reid described transvaginal ultrasonography with a rigid transducer in 1957. This type of transducer was, however, never used in clinical practice. With the development of high-frequency transvaginal transducers in 1983, ultrasound became an important tool in the diagnosis of early pregnancy.[26–27] The gestation sac can be visualized from around 36 days from the last menstrual period (LMP), when it reaches a size of 2–4 mm, corresponding to a level of hCG of 800 to 3200 IU/L.[28] The yolk sac can be observed when the gestational sac exceeds 10 mm.[11,29] Once the gestation sac reaches 20 mm, the embryo should be identified.[30,31] One-third of normal viable embryos with a crown–rump length (CRL) of less than 5 mm have no demonstrable cardiac activity. Therefore, repeated scanning with an interval of a few days is necessary before the definite diagnosis of non-viable pregnancy is made.[32] We know that a small or irregular gestational

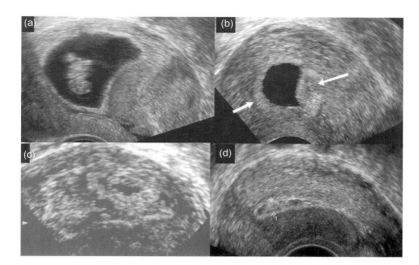

Figure 5.1 Four different ultrasound classifications of miscarriage: (a) early fetal demise (formally missed miscarriage); (b) early embryonic demise (formally blighted ovum or anembryonic pregnancy); (c) incomplete miscarriage; (d) 'complete miscarriage' should now be included under the umbrella term 'pregnancy of unknown location'.

sac, discrepancies between the CRL and pregnancy length and an abnormal pattern of embryonic heart rate are predictors of a poor pregnancy outcome.[31,33] The presence of subchorionic bleeding per se does not seem to be a negative prognostic sign, unless it is located at the level of the definitive placenta, i.e. under the cord insertion.[31,34] The absence of an intrauterine gestational sac when hCG levels are above 1000 IU/L is highly suspicious of an ectopic pregnancy.[29,35]

In cases of non-viability, ultrasound allows us to evaluate the amount of retained products of conception in the uterus and thus may lead to an avoidance of unnecessary intervention in apparent complete miscarriages.[19,36–38] In cases of miscarriage, it is possible to differentiate roughly between four different ultrasound features:

1. 'Intra-uterine fetal demise', also called 'missed miscarriage' (Figure 5.1a).
2. 'Embryonic demise', also called 'blighted ovum', characterized by an empty gestational sac (Figure 5.1b), or 'anembryonic pregnancy'.
3. 'Complex mass', characterized by areas of different echogenicity caused by bleeding in the gestational sac (Figure 5.1c). This is known as an incomplete miscarriage.
4. Finally 'complete miscarriage' (Figure 5.1d), where an empty uterine cavity is noted or

where there is only a minimal, non-significant amount of retained products with an antero-posterior diameter less than 15 mm in the longitudinal view of the uterus. The antero-posterior diameter is measured in between the myometrium and endometrium border as shown in Figure 5.1b.

The term should now be included under the umbrella term 'pregnancy of unknown location'.

In first trimester pregnancies an acellular fluid occupies the intervillous space. An increase in the placental blood flow in complicated pregnancies compared with normal pregnancies has been shown with Doppler ultrasound.[39] This also correlates with histopathological findings suggesting that miscarriage begins with dislocation and disruption of the trophoblastic shell with premature entry of maternal blood into the intervillous space.[31] It is possible that blood flow patterns in the intervillous space, demonstrated by Doppler ultrasound, could be used to forecast the outcome of expectant management of miscarriage.[40,41]

TREATMENT OF MISCARRIAGE

A historical perspective

In an analysis of 2287 cases of miscarriage including an unknown number of illegal abortions registered in Baltimore from 1896 to

1934, the average pregnancy length was 14 weeks measured from the LMP.[42] Only women who were bleeding excessively or had infections were admitted to the hospital. Over 50% of those women had a gestation of above 16 weeks. The mortality was 1.7% in this cohort of women and the majority of deaths were attributed to infections, and in no instance was haemorrhage the immediate cause of death. The true number of criminal or illegal abortions was unknown, but 9% of the women admitted to having undergone such a procedure.

In the 1930s Collins managed 1304 cases of miscarriage medically with oxytocics. There were six deaths due to infection.[43] He described 14 additional deaths during an earlier period with only one death due to haemorrhage, the rest being due to infections. Roussel treated 3739 cases of miscarriage between 1933 and 1944 with oxytocics and reported an average hospital stay of 14 days. There were 51 deaths, ten of them because of blood loss and the rest mainly again because of infection.[12] It is reasonable to conclude that prior to the antibiotic era, infection and not haemorrhage was the predominant threat to women undergoing miscarriage.

To prevent miscarriage and other pregnancy problems such as toxaemia, premature delivery and intrauterine fetal death, about six million pregnant women were exposed to diethylstilboestrol (DES) from 1940 until 1971. Fortunately, some of the users were included in controlled studies that showed that DES was of no value to prevent miscarriage, or in preventing any of the other conditions for which it was given. On the contrary, DES carried an increased risk of the patients' developing breast cancer, and for the offspring a higher risk of genitourinary malformations, psychiatric disorders and vaginal or cervical clear cell adenocarcinoma.[44–47]

In 2665 women treated surgically with a presumed diagnosis of miscarriage between 1934 and 1949 the mortality rate was 0.26%.[13] Compared to historical controls, this mortality rate seemed to be low, indicating that active treatment was more effective than conservative management. In this study, the author had the impression that 90% of the miscarriages were in fact criminal abortions. Most of the severe complications were following douching, during which fluid was forcibly flushed into the uterine cavity. All the deaths were due to infection.[13] Soap bubble embolism was assumed to be the cause of some cases of sudden death, but these women never arrived at the hospital.[31] In a survey in 1950 of 727 incomplete miscarriages treated actively by curettage, the women had an average hospital stay of 4.8 days with no mortality reported.[48] This was a superior figure compared to women managed conservatively.[31] It is, however, difficult to compare these four studies since penicillin, which came into use in 1945, was not available to Pecham's, Roussel's or Collins' cases, and morbidity and mortality was mainly related to sepsis. It is not surprising that surgical evacuation under these circumstances was seen as an adequate and sometimes life-saving treatment for women with symptoms of miscarriage, especially when criminal abortion could not be ruled out. Hertig and Livingston stated in 1944 that the treatment of miscarriage was a matter of emptying the uterus as quickly and as safely as possible. This general consensus prevailed for the last five decades concerning the superiority of surgical evacuation in cases of miscarriage.[49–51]

Current management

The majority of miscarriages are today diagnosed in the first trimester, and illegal abortion is almost an unknown phenomenon in the majority of industrialized nations.[10] Despite these changes, routine surgical evacuation has remained the treatment of choice in cases of miscarriage. In the early 1990s surgical evacuation of miscarriages accounted for about three-quarters of 'out of office time' surgical interventions in gynaecological practice in Britain.[50] The justification for surgical evacuation in cases of miscarriage has been the concern that retained products of conception within the uterus might lead to infection or haemorrhage.[51]

Surgery

There is today an increasing awareness that surgical evacuation of the uterine cavity during early pregnancy has risks and may cause seque-lae. Infection, secondary infertility, dyspareunia and chronic pelvic pain have been associated with overt and subclinical infections after evacuations for legal terminations.[52] In 111 women treated by suction curettage for miscarriage, Farrel and co-workers observed a complication rate of 9%, and half of the complications were directly related to the surgical procedure.[53] In women treated for first trimester miscarriage, Hinshaw and co-workers found pelvic inflammatory disease in 13.2% of women treated by suction curettage and 7.1% of women treated medically (P <0.001).[54] During the last few years, the use of misoprostol in cases of illegal abortion has become a common method of pregnancy termination in Brazil. Interestingly, the rate of infection after illegal abortions has decreased from 49% after invasive methods to 4% following misoprostol.[15,55] On the other hand, it is important to point out that teratogenic effects of misoprostol have been reported in cases of unsuccessful termination.[56]

Surgical evacuation is also associated with rare but serious morbidity such as uterine perforation, bowel damage and anaesthetic risks. Following legal abortions performed through surgical evacuation an incidence of serious morbidity of 2.1% and a mortality of 0.5 per 100 000 have been demonstrated.[57]

Medical management

During the last decade, early termination of pregnancy with the anti-progesterone mifepristone in combination with prostaglandins has become a common treatment. Several hundred anti-progestins have been synthesized, but only mifepristone, lilopristone (ZK 98.734) and onapristone (ZK 98.299) have been given to humans.[58] Most of the clinical research to date has focused on the use of mifepristone given in combination with prostaglandin analogues. Mifepristone is a steroid hormone antagonist with a high affinity to progesterone and gluco-corticoid receptors.[59] There are two main types of progesterone receptors; type A and type B. These receptors can form homo- or hetero-dimers, both of which can interact with the same DNA sequence.[60] Mifepristone mediates the antagonistic effect by binding to the type A progesterone receptor. In the absence of progesterone receptor A, antagonist-occupied receptor B dimers can promote transcription without binding of the progesterone receptor to DNA. A lack of response to progesterone antagonists has been observed in chickens and progesterone receptor mutation in humans has been suggested to be responsible for the unresponsiveness to mifepristone in some women.[61]

Mifepristone blocks progesterone receptors in the endometrium. This causes vascular damage, which prevents decidualization, followed by decidual necrosis and development of uterine contractions with detachment of products of conception.[62,63] Prostaglandins stimulate the contractility of the myometrium and blockade of the progesterone receptor by mifepristone increases the sensitivity of the myometrium to prostaglandins and oxytocin.[63–65] A dose-dependent stimulation of prostaglandin $F_{2\alpha}$ and prostaglandin E_2 synthesis by mifepristone has been demonstrated in human endometrial and decidual cell cultures.[66] When mifepristone is administered to pregnant women prior to termination of pregnancy it softens the cervix and increases the uterine contractile activity.[67,68] The effect of mifepristone on the pregnant cervix seems not to be mediated through an increased production of prostaglandins.[69]

In cases of legal termination, treatment with mifepristone alone results in a high rate of incomplete abortions, suggesting that the release of prostaglandins is inadequate.[65,70] The success rate in cases of termination has been found to be maximized when prostaglandin analogues are administered 36–48 hours after mifepristone.[71] Thong and Baird demonstrated that mifepristone 200 mg in combination with misoprostol 600 µg resulted in complete abortion in 92% of women applying for termination before 56 days of amenorrhoea (8 weeks).[72] Pharmacological treatment is today an accepted alternative to surgical termination. During the last few years pharmacological treatment has also been proposed as an alternative to surgical evacuation in cases of miscarriage.[64,73–76] Misoprostol alone has been used in total doses from 600 µg with success rates ranging from 13% to close to 100%. In all these trials the women have been hospitalised or managed in a day-care setting.[73–75,77] Since our study from 1995 demonstrated that almost 80% of the women achieved a complete miscarriage within 3 days of expectant management, these results are difficult to interpret.[78] Misoprostol is a potent prostaglandin analogue with well-known side effects such as severe pain and gastrointestinal symptoms. While doses of 400 µg are relatively well tolerated by pregnant women, doses above 400 µg necessitate hospitalization to relieve side effects.[73,74,77,79] In cases of legal abortion, prostaglandin E_2 given in clinically acceptable doses has not been effective enough to induce termination.[65]

Sulprostone, gemeprost and misoprostol have been the most frequently used prostaglandin analogues. Sulprostone, a prostaglandin E_2 analogue given intramuscularly, has proved to give cardiovascular complications and is therefore no longer in use. Although slightly less effective when compared with gemeprost (prostaglandin E_1 vaginal suppository), misoprostol (a prostaglandin E_1 analogue) is easier to use, less expensive and does not require special storage conditions.[54,72,79,80]

Methotrexate, an analogue of folic acid that inhibits the production of folates required for de novo purine and pyrimidine synthesis, prevents cell division. Methotrexate is also directly cytotoxic to both neoplastic and non-neoplastic trophoblastic tissue. Methotrexate has been used to terminate early ectopic pregnancy since the early 1980s and in combination with misoprostol for legal terminations in Canada and the USA since 1993.[81–84] In spite of the fact that methotrexate is highly effective in inhibiting trophoblastic proliferation, it has not been reported to have been used for the treatment of miscarriages.

Mifepristone and misoprostol have been proposed for the pharmacological treatment of miscarriages and early fetal demise (missed miscarriage/blighted ovum). The use of misoprostol alone in repeated doses from 400 µg orally, has succeeded in avoiding surgery in 95% of women with first-trimester incomplete miscarriage.[64,73,76,77,85] Nielsen and co-workers (1998) avoided surgery in 81% of the women with first-trimester miscarriage using misoprostol 400 µg orally.[96] Chung and co-workers, using misoprostol 400 µg t.i.d. orally, avoided surgery in 85% of women with first trimester incomplete miscarriage.[73] In another trial, the same authors, extending the use of misoprostol to 48 hours, avoided surgery in 148 of 225 women (65%) with incomplete miscarriage.[74] De Jonge and co-workers tested 400 µg of misoprostol orally with an end-point at 12 hours and avoided surgery in only 13% of incomplete miscarriages.[75]

Early fetal or embryonic demise has also been treated pharmacologically by Lelaider and co-workers who avoided surgery in 17 of 23 cases of missed miscarriage with mifepristone 600 mg.[85] El-Refay and co-workers succeeded in avoiding surgery in 54 of 59 cases of missed miscarriage using a combination of 600 mg of mifepristone followed by 600 µg of misoprostol orally.[77]

The results of these studies are somewhat confusing, with success rates varying from 13 to 95%, which probably is due to different inclusion criteria. As we will discuss later, in many of these cases the miscarriages would have resolved without any intervention at all and success related to the case mix. In addition, in all these studies the women were dependent on hospitalization in order to relieve side effects related to the relatively high doses of misoprostol given. Besides operating theatre time, hospitalization accounts for the largest part of the costs connected with the treatment of miscarriage.[86]

More recently it has been shown that prior to miscarriage there is an increase in nitric oxide release and that this may contribute to cervical ripening and the onset of clinical miscarriage. This opens new therapeutic possibilities to women with missed miscarriages and incomplete miscarriage who do not resolve in a short period of time.[87]

EXPECTANT MANAGEMENT OF MISCARRIAGE

For many years there was a consensus that prevailed in the Western world concerning the approach to miscarriages and custom has dictated that inevitable and incomplete miscarriages must be completed, usually by curettage. Many physicians considered curettage mandatory to prove that a miscarriage is complete. Expectant management of first-trimester miscarriages had not been evaluated since Peckham stated in 1936 that women without profuse bleeding or signs of infection could avoid hospitalization.[42] The justification for surgical evacuation as the correct management of first-trimester miscarriages was based on case reports and uncontrolled studies from a time when general health, parity, availability of health services, antibiotics and the incidence of criminal abortions differed greatly from now. The consensus has changed during the last decade and expectant management as well as different medical regimens for the conservative management of miscarriage have been evaluated.

In a randomized study between expectant management and surgical evacuation in 1995, of 103 women randomized to expectant management spontaneous resolution of the pregnancy products occurred within 3 days in 81 cases (79%). The remaining women underwent surgical evacuation.[78]

In another study 545 women with a diagnosis of early pregnancy failure were followed up; 298 with incomplete miscarriage and 247 with missed miscarriage or anembryonic pregnancies. A total of 305 of them opted for expectant management. The overall success rate was of 86%. The success rate for incomplete miscarriage (96%) was significantly better than that for missed miscarriage (62%).[88] In 2002 Luise and co-workers presented a comparative study between expectant management and surgical evacuation. They found a resolution rate after 14 days of 84%; they also found that neither the presence of a gestational sac, nor the endometrial thickness at diagnosis can be used to predict the likelihood of management failure.[89] According to the data of Nielsen and Hahlin there is a significant correlation between levels of S-progesterone and hCG and the success rate of expectant management.[90] In this study utilizing a stepwise logistic regression procedure, five diagnostic variables possessing prognostic power were identified: serum progesterone, daily serum hCG change, serum CA125, serum alpha fetoprotein and intrauterine diameter. The logistic regression analysis was also applied to three diagnostic variables chosen for routine clinical use: serum progesterone, serum hCG and intrauterine diameter. Using this algorithm, the probability of complete spontaneous miscarriage within 3 days of expectant management in each woman could be calculated. It was concluded that a logistic model to calculate the probability of complete spontaneous miscarriage within 3 days in women with first-trimester miscarriages is effective. Such information may be of clinical use in caring for women, as well as for the development of management guidelines for those with miscarriages.[90]

The complication rate, most commonly infection and haemorrhage, reported after surgical evacuation in cases of miscarriage and legal abortion varies between 4 and 13%.[53,54,91,92] Infections after surgical evacuation are often easily treated but may lead to infertility, pelvic pain and an increased risk of future ectopic pregnancy.[74,91] Dilatation of the cervical canal may interfere with the cervical protection against ascending infections, whilst curettage carries the risk of contaminating the uterine cavity.[91] These risks of introducing an infection by surgical evacuation should be weighed against the possible hazards of leaving retained products of conception in the uterine cavity for long periods of time.

In a study by Nielsen and Hahlin only three infections were diagnosed among 103 women (3%) who underwent expectant management.[78] In comparison, five infections and one case of postoperative anaemia were observed among 52 women (11%) randomized to surgical evacuation.[78] In another study presented by the same group three infections were reported amongst 122 women primarily managed non-surgically.[86] Interestingly, infections in this study were only diagnosed among women who underwent surgery due to retained products of conception 5 days after inclusion.[86] All women were followed up with serum samples and clinical examination 3 or 5 and 14 days after inclusion. It is possible that many infections which otherwise would have passed without intervention were discovered and treated because of the close follow-up in the study. On the other hand, 'sub-clinical' infections after a miscarriage may carry the risk of sequelae such as infertility and chronic pain.[91] The mean time during which the women experienced vaginal bleeding was 1.3 days longer in the expectant management group compared to the group who underwent surgical evacuation.[86] This is probably due to a quicker resolution of the retained products of conception for the women randomized to surgical evacuation.

Medical management of miscarriage

Hughes and co-workers, who compared women treated medically and surgically, observed 7.1% infections in women managed medically compared to 13.2% in women managed surgically (P <0.001, χ^2).[93] These studies may suggest that surgical evacuation of the uterine cavity in early pregnancy carries an increased risk of PID compared to non-surgical management.

Medical treatment for miscarriage with prostaglandins alone or in combination with the antiprogesterone mifepristone has been explored. There are a few randomized studies comparing expectant with medical management, the success rate varies probably due to different doses and inclusion criteria.[86,94–96] It seems, however, that medical treatment is slightly more effective than expectant management alone. Treatment with misoprostol is potentially dangerous to a normal ongoing pregnancy, due to its abortifacient effect and teratogenicity. Careful assessment with an exact diagnosis is mandatory before treatment with misoprostol. This is not always available at an emergency room. In addition it seems that medical treatment is accompanied with more pain than expectant management. It would therefore seem reasonable to propose a strategy whereby misoprostol could be used as second line treatment after an initial attempt to manage things expectantly for at least a week.[95] In this way intervention may be avoided in the majority of women where the miscarriage will resolve spontaneously.[86,95,96] One should also bear in mind that most women with retained products of conception will probably chose expectant

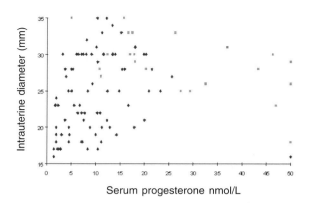

Figure 5.2 Relationship between sac volume and serum progesterone.

management. Furthermore, ultrasonography can be used to advise women on the likelihood that their miscarriage will complete spontaneously within a given time. Fifty-two per cent of incomplete miscarriages will resolve spontaneously by day 7 of management and 84% by day 14. Furthermore, the corresponding values for missed miscarriages and anembryonic pregnancies are 28% by day 7 and 56% by day 14.[89] This means that most women who miscarry in the first trimester and choose expectant management will complete their miscarriage without intervention.

Ultrasonography provides a useful assessment of whether a miscarriage will complete without intervention within a given time. The first randomized study exploring expectant management for miscarriage[78] excluded women with an antero-posterior diameter of retained products of conception in uterus of >50 mm and all studies since then have used similar cut-off values on the assumption that larger amounts of retained products of conception will be followed by more bleeding and pain. The relationship between volume and serum progesterone and diameter and the outcome of expectant management of 103 women managed expectantly is illustrated in Figure 5.2. Blue dots represent women who miscarried without intervention within three days of expectant management. Diameters in the antero-posterior view of retained products in uterus bellow 15 mm have been considered as being consistent with a complete miscarriage. This is also supported by an analysis of 118 women followed up after a complete miscarriage (diameter <15 mm) where none were admitted for surgical intervention after the first visit.[98] As discussed in other chapters, the ultrasound findings are not sufficient to confirm a complete miscarriage, and serial hCG levels are needed to exclude an ectopic pregnancy in these women.

Available data show that expectant management for the majority of women with first-trimester miscarriage is a safe procedure. Furthermore, available data today suggest that the complication rate, fertility,[99] and the emotional and psychological short-term complications[100,101] do not differ significantly between different treatment modalities for miscarriage.

CONCLUSIONS

We believe that TVS can be used to advise women of the likelihood that their miscarriage will complete spontaneously within given periods of time from the day of classification. However, there still is a need for further studies to enable the identification of those women who are unlikely to complete their miscarriage spontaneously, and to determine the relative efficacy rates and side effects of alternative treatments. Furthermore, we emphasize the importance of providing information to the woman regarding all treatment options.

CASE REPORT

A 29-year-old woman presented to the Early Pregnancy Unit at 10^{+4} weeks' gestation in her first pregnancy. She was complaining of light vaginal bleeding and cramp-like lower abdominal pain. A transvaginal ultrasound scan was performed which showed an empty intrauterine gestational sac measuring $24 \times 26 \times 23$ mm. A diagnosis of delayed miscarriage (or blighted ovum) was made. Conservative and surgical management options were discussed, but she decided to be managed expectantly. She returned to the Early Pregnancy Unit 1 week later for review with a history of increased vaginal bleeding. A repeat scan showed retained products of conception measuring $20 \times 18 \times 21$ mm. She was re-scanned a week later and was confirmed as having had a complete miscarriage, with an endometrial thickness of 8 mm with no evidence of retained products of conception.

PRACTICAL POINTS

1. Arrangements to provide information, follow-up, counselling and support by dedicated personnel for women with first trimester miscarriages should be made in all departments of obstetrics and gynaecology. These departments should formulate guidelines for the management of first trimester miscarriage and provide access to specialized personnel familiar with the use of transvaginal ultrasound in early pregnancy.
2. Expectant management should be considered for all women presenting with symptoms of an incomplete miscarriage.
3. Complete miscarriage cannot be diagnosed with confidence by ultrasonography. If there is no tissue in the endometrial cavity the women must be managed as a PUL as there is a risk of ectopic pregnancy.
4. Medical pharmacological treatment with adequate doses of prostaglandin analogues have a place in the treatment of certain women with inevitable miscarriage and early fetal demise.

REFERENCES

1. Hegar A. Diagnose der frühesten Schwangerschaftsperiode. Deutsche medisinsche wochenschrift 1895; 35:564–72.

2. Aschheim S, Zondek B. Hyppofysenwordenlappen hormon und ovarialhormon im Harm von Schangeren. Klinisch Wochenschrift 1927; 6:1322.

3. Wide L, Gemzell CA. An immunological pregnancy test. Acta Endocr 1960; 35:261–4.

4. Roberts CJ, Lowe CR. Where have all the conceptions gone? Lancet 1975; 1:498–500.

5. Miller JF, Williamson E, Glue J, Gordon YB, Grudzinskas JG, Sykes A. Fetal loss after implantation. A prospective study. Lancet, 1980; 2:554–6.

6. Tietze C, Guttmacher AF, Rubin S. Unintentional abortion in 1497 planned pregnancies. JAMA 1950; 142:1348–50.

7. Laferla JJ. Spontaneous abortion. Clin Obstet Gynaecol 1986; 13:105–14.

8. Hammerslough CR. Estimating the probability of spontaneous abortion in the presence of induced abortion and vice versa. Public Health Reports 1992; 107:269–77.

9. Prendiville WJ. Miscarriage: epidemiological aspects. In: Grudzinskas JG, O'Brian PMS, eds. Problems in early pregnancy: Advances in diagnosis and management. RCOG Press 1997; 3–18.

10. Brambati B. Fate of human pregnancie. Establishing a successful human pregnancy. Serono symposia 1990; 66:269–81. New York: Raven Press.

11. Goldstein SR. Sonography in early pregnancy failure. Clin Obstet Gynecol 1994; 37:681–92.

12. Roussel PB. Abortion treated conservatively. A 12-year study covering 3739 cases. South M J 1947; 40:314 255–63.

13. Davis A. Clinical survey of 2665 cases of abortions. BMJ 1950; 2:123–30.

14. Dutra FR, Cleveland FP, Lyle HP. Criminal abortions induced by intrauterine pastes. JAMA 1950; 143:865–9.

15. Facundes A, Santos LC, Carvalho M, Gras C. Post-abortion complications after interruption of pregnancy with misoprostol. Adv Contracept 1996; 12:1–9.

16. Rees H, Katzenellenbogen J, Shabodien R, Fawcus S, McIntyre J, Lombard C, Truter H. The epidemiology of incomplete abortion in South Africa. National Incomplete Abortion Reference Group. S Afr Med J 1997; 87:417–18.

17. Cook RJ, Dickens BM, Bliss LE. International developments in abortion law from 1988 to 1998. Am J Public Health 1999; 89(4):579–86.

18. Bastian LA, Piscitelli JT. Is this patient pregnant? Can you reliably rule in or rule out early pregnancy by clinical examination? JAMA 1997; 278:586–91.

19. Hahlin M, Thorburn J, Bryman I. The expectant management of early pregnancies of uncertain site. Hum Reprod 1995; 10:1223–7.

20. Dilts PV Jr. Abnormalities and complications of pregnancy. Spontaneous abortion. The Merk Manual 14th edition, 1982, pp. 1723–5.

21. Hagström HG, Hahlin M, Sjöblom P, Lindblom B. Prediction of persistent trophoblastic activity after local prostaglandin $F_{2\alpha}$ injection for ectopic pregnancy. Hum Reprod 1994; 9:1170–4.

22. Gelder MS, Boots LR, Younger JB. Use of a single random serum progesterone value as a diagnostic aid for ectopic pregnancy. Fert Steril 1991; 55:497–500.

23. Lindblom B, Hahlin M, Sjöblom P. Serial human chorionic gonadotropin determinations by fluoroimmunoassay for differentiation between intrauterine and ectopic gestation. Am J Obstet Gynecol 1989; 161:397–400.

24. Hagström HG, Hahlin M, Bennegård-Eden B, Sjöblom P, Thorburn J, Lindblom B. Prediction of persistent ectopic pregnancy after laparoscopic salpingostomy. Obstet Gynecol 1994; 5:798–802.

25. Elson J, Jurkovic D. Biochemistry in diagnosis and management of abnormal early pregnancy. Curr Opin Obstet Gynecol 2004; 16(4):339–44.

26. Schwimer S, Lebovic J. Transvaginal pelvic ultrasonography. J Ultrasound Med 1984; 3:381–3.

27. Wikland M, Hamberger L. Transvesical and transvaginal approaches for aspiration of follicles by use of ultrasound. Ann NY Acad Sci 1985; 442:182–94.

28. Bateman BG, Nunley WC Jr, Kolp LA, Kitchin JD, Felder R. Vaginal sonography findings and hCG dynamics of early intrauterine and tubal pregnancies. Obstet Gynecol 1990; 75:421–7.

29. Cacciatore B, Pekka Y, Stenman UH, Widholm O. Suspected ectopic pregnancy: ultrasound findings and hCG levels assesed by an immunofluorometric assay. Br J Obstet Gynecol 1988; 95:497–502.

30. Cacciatore B, Tiitinen A, Stenman UH, Ylöstalo P. Normal early pregnancy: serum levels and vaginal ultrasonography findings. Br J Obstet Gynecol 1990; 97:899–903.

31. Jauniaux E, Zaidi J, Jurkovic D, Campbell S, Hustin J. Comparison of colour doppler features and pathological findings in complicated early pregnancy. Hum Reprod 1994; 9:2432–7.

32. Hately W, Case J, Campbell S. Establishing the death of an embryo by ultrasound: report of a public inquiry with recommendations. Ultrasound Obstet Gynecol 1995; 5:353–7.

33. Martinez JM, Comas C, OJuel J, et al. Fetal heart rate patterns in pregnancies with chromosomal disorders or subsequent fetal loss. Obstet Gynecol 1996; 87:118–21.

34. Ball RH, Ade CM, Schoenborn JA, Crane JP. The clini-

cal significance of ultransonographically detected subchorionic hemorrhages. Am J Obstet Gynecol 1996; 174:996–1002.

35. Enk L, Wikland M, Hammarberg K, Lindblom B. The value of endovaginal sonography and urinary human chorionic gonadotrophin test for the differentiation between intrauterine and ectopic pregnancy. J Clin Ultrasound 1990; 18:73–8.

36. Haines CH, Chung T, Leung DYL. Transvaginal sonography and the conservative management of spontaneous abortion. Gynecol Obstet Invest 1994; 37:14–17.

37. Mansur MM. Ultrasound diagnosis of complete abortion can reduce need for curettage. Eur Obstet Gynecol Reprod Biol 1992; 44:65–9.

38. Rulin MC, Bornstein SG, Campell JD. The reliability of ultrasonography in the management of spontaneous abortion, clinically thought to be complete: A prospective study. Am J Obstet Gynecol 1993; 168:12–15.

39. Jaffe R, Dorgan A, Abramowicz JS. Color Doppler imaging of the uteroplacental circulation in the first trimester: value in predicting pregnancy failure or complication. Am J Roentgenol 1995; 164:1255–8.

40. Schwarzler P, Holden D, Nielsen S, et al. The conservative management of first trimester miscarriages and the use of colour Doppler sonography for patient selection. Hum Reprod 1999; 14(5):1341–5.

41. Alcazar JL, Ortiz CA. Transvaginal color Doppler ultrasonography in the management of first-trimester spontaneous abortion. Eur J Obstet Gynecol Reprod Biol 2002; 102(1):83–7.

42. Peckham CH, Abortion: A statistical analysis of 2287 Cases. Surg Gynecol Obstet 1936; 63:204–63.

43. Collins JH. Abortions – a study based on 1304 cases. Am J Obst Gynecol 1951; 62:213–16.

44. Beral V, Colwell L. Randomised trial of high doses of stilboestrol and ethisterone therapy in pregnancy: long-term follow-up of the children. J Epidemiol Comm Health 1981; 35:155–60.

45. Vessey MP, Fairweather DV, Norman-Smith B, Buckley J. A randomized double-blind controlled trial of the value of stilboestrol therapy in pregnancy: long-term follow-up of mothers and their offspring. Br J Obstet Gynaecol 1983; 90:1007–17.

46. Monaghan JM, Sirisena LA. Stilboestrol and vaginal clear-cell adenocarcinoma syndrome. BMJ 1978; 1:1588–90.

47. Salle B, Sergeant P, Awada A, et al. Transvaginal ultrasound studies of vascular and morphological changes in uteri exposed to diethylstilbestrol in utero. Hum Reprod 1996 11:2531–6.

48. Greenhill JP, ed. Year book of obstetrics and gynecology. 1951: 39–41.

49. Peretz A, Grunstein S, Brandes JM, Paldi E. Evacuation of the gravid uterus by negative pressure (suction evacuation). Am J Obstet Gynecol 1967; 98(1): 18–22

50. McKee M, Priest P, Ginzlet M, Black N. Can out-of-hours operating in gynaecology be reduced? Arch Emerg Med 1992; 9:290–8.

51. Huisjes HJ. Spontaneous abortion. Current reviews in obstetrics and gynaecology. Vol 8. Edinburgh: Churchill Livingstone 1984.

52. Heisterberg L, Hebjörn S, Andersen LF, Petersen H. Sequelae of induced first-trimester abortion. A prospective study assessing the role of postabortal pelvic inflammatory disease and prophylactic antibiotics. Am J Obstet Gynecol 1986; 155:76–80.

53. Farell RG, Stonington DT, Ridgeway RA. Incomplete and inevitable abortion: Treatment by suction curettage in the emergency department. Ann Emerg Med 1982; 11:652–8.

54. Hinshaw HK. Medical management of miscarriage. In: Grudzinskas JG, O'Brian PMS, eds. Problems in early pregnancy: Advances in diagnosis and management. RCOG Press 1997; 284–95.

55. Costa SH, Vessey MP. Misoprostol and illegal abortion in Rio de Janeiro, Brazil. Lancet 1993; 341:1258–61.

56. Gonzalez CH, Vargas FR, Perez AB, et al. Limb deficiency with or without Möbius sequence in seven Brazilian children associated with misoprostol use in the first trimester of pregnancy. Am J Med Genet 1993; 47:59–64.

57. Lawson HW, Frye A, Atrash HK, et al. Abortion mortality, United States, 1872 through 1987. Am J Obstet Gynecol 1994; 171:1365–72.

58. Van Look PF, von Hertzen H. Clinical uses of antiprogestogens. Hum Reprod Update 1995; 1:19–34.

59. Baulieu EE. On the mechanism of action of RU 486. Frontiers in human reproduction. Ann NY Acad Sci 1991; 626:545–60.

60. Pinter JH, Dee PC, Ok-Yong PS. Progesterone receptors: expression and regulation in the mammalian ovary. Clin Obst Gynaecol 1996; 39:424–35.

61. Johanisson E, Oberholzer M, Swhan ML, Bygdeman M. Vascular changes in the human endometrium following the administration of the progesterone antagonist RU 486. Contraception 1989; 39:103–17.

62. Bygdeman M, Gemzell K, Gottlieb C, Swahn ML. Uterine contractility and interaction between prostaglandins and antiprogestins. Clinical implications. Ann NY Acad Sci 1991; 626:561–7. Review.

63. Bygdeman M, Swahn ML, Gemzell-Danielsson K, Svalander P. Mode of action of RU 486. Ann Med 1993; 25:61–4.

64. Bygdeman M, Swahn ML, Gemzell-Danielsson K, Gottlieb C. The use of progesterone antagonists in combination with prostaglandin for termination of pregnancy. Hum Reprod 1994; 9:121–5.

65. Swahn ML, Gottlieb C, Green K, Bygdeman M. Oral administration of RU 486 and 9-methylene PGE2 for termination of early pregnancy. Contraception 1990; 41:461–73.

66. Smith SK, Kelly RW. The effect of the antiprogestins RU 486 and ZK 98734 on the synthesis and metabolism of prostaglandin F_2 alpha and E_2 in separated cells from early human decidua. J Clin Endocrinol Metab 1987; 65:527–34.

67. Rådestad A, Bygdeman M, Green K. Induced cervical ripening with mifepristone (RU 486) and bioconversion of arachidonic acid in human pregnant uterine cervix in the first trimester. A double blind randomized biomechanical and biochemical study. Contraception 1990; 41:283–92.

68. Bygdeman M, Swahn ML. Progesterone receptor blockage. Effect on uterine contractility and early pregnancy. Contraception 1985; 32:45–51.

69. Rådestad A, Bygdeman M. Cervical softening with mifepristone (RU 486) after pretreatment with naproxen. A double-blind randomized study. Contraception 1992; 45:221–7.

70. Grimes DA, Mishell DR Jr, David HP. A randomised clinical trial of mifepristone (RU 486) for induction of delayed menses: efficacy and acceptability. Contraception 1992; 46:1–10.

71. Ulmann A, Silvestre L, Chemama L, et al. Medical termination of early pregnancy with mifepristone followed by a prostaglandin analogue: study in 16,369 women. Acta Obstet Gynecol Scand 1992;71:278–83.

72. Thong KJ, Baird DT. Induction of abortion with mifepristone and misoprostol in early pregnancy. Br J Obstet Gynaecol 1992; 99:1004–7.

73. Chung TK, Cheung LP, Leung TY, Haines CJ, Chang AM. Misoprostol in the management of spontaneous abortion. Br J Obstet Gynaecol 1995; 102:832–5.

74. Chung TK, Leung P, Cheung LP, Haines C, Chang AM. A medical approach to management of spontaneous abortion using misoprostol. Extending misoprostol treatment to a maximum of 48 hours can further improve evacuation of retained products of conception in spontaneous abortion. Acta Obstet Gynecol Scand 1997; 76(3):248–51.

75. De Jonge ET, Makin JD, Manefeldt E, De Wet GH, Pattinson RC. Randomised clinical trial of medical evacuation and surgical curettage for incomplete miscarriage. BMJ 1995; 311:662.

76. Henshaw RC, Cooper K, El-Refaey H, Smith NC, Templeton AA. Medical management of miscarriage: non-surgical uterine evacuation of incomplete and inevitable spontaneous abortion. BMJ 1993; 306:894–5.

77. El-Refaey H, Hinshaw K, Henshaw R, Smith N, Tempelton A. Medical management of missed abortion and anembryonic pregnancy BMJ 1992; 305:1399.

78. Nielsen S, Hahlin M. Expectant management of first-trimester spontaneous abortion. Lancet 1995; 345(8942):84–6.

79. Platz-Christensen JJ, Nielsen S, Hamberger L. Is misoprostol the drug of choice for induced cervical ripening in early pregnancy termination? Acta Obstet Gynecol Scand 1995; 74:809–12.

80. Peplow PV. RU486 combined with PGE_1 analog in voluntary termination of early pregnancy: a comparison of recent findings with gemeprost or misoprostol. Contraception 1994; 50:69–75.

81. Bengtsson G, Bryman I, Thorburn J, Lindblom B. Low-dose oral methotrexate as second-line therapy for persistent trophoblast after conservative treatment of ectopic pregnancy. Obstet Gynecol 1992; 79:589–91.

82. Stoval TG, Ling FW. Single-dose methotrexate: an expanded clinical trial. Am J Obstet Gynecol 1993; 168:1759–65.

83. Creinin MD, Vittinghoff E, Keder L, Darney PD, Tiller G. Methotrexate and misoprostol for early abortion: a multicenter trial: safety and efficacy. Contraception 1996; 53:321–7.

84. Creinin MD, Krohn MA. Methotrexate pharmacokinetics and effects in women receiving methotrexate 50 mg and 60 mg per square meter for early abortion. Am J Ostet Gynecol 1997; 177:1444–9.

85. Lelaider C, Baton-Saint-Mleux C, Fernandez H, Bourget P, Frydman R. Mifepristone (RU 486) induces expulsion in first trimester non-developing pregnancies: a prospective randomised trial. Hum Reprod 1993; 8:492–5.

86. Nielsen S, Hahlin M, Platz-Christensen J. Randomised trial comparing expectant with medical management for first trimester miscarriages. Br J Obstet Gynaecol 1999; 106(8):804–7.

87. Vaisanen-Tommiska M, Mikkola TS, Ylikorkala O. Increased release of cervical nitric oxide in spontaneous abortion before clinical symptoms: a possible mechanism for preabortal cervical ripening. J Clin Endocrinol Metab 2004; 89(11):5622–6.

88. Sairam S, Khare M, Michailidis G, Thilaganathan B. The role of ultrasound in the expectant management of early pregnancy loss. Ultrasound Obstet Gynecol 2001; 17:506–9.

89. Luise C, Jermy K, May C, et al. Outcome of expectant management of spontaneous first trimester miscarrige: observational study. BMJ 2002; 324:873–5.

90. Nielsen S, Hahlin M, Oden A. Using a logistic model to identify women with first-trimester spontaneous abortion suitable for expectant management. Br J Obstet Gynaecol 1997; 104(6):755–6.

91. Heisterberg L, Kringelbach M. Early complications after induced first-trimester abortion. Acta Obstet Gynecol Scand 1987; 66:201–4.

92. Laferla JJ. Spontaneous abortion. Clin Obstet Gynaecol 1986; 13:105–14.

93. Hughes J, Ryan M, Hinshaw K, et al. The costs of treating miscarriage: a comparison of medical and surgical management. Br J Obstet Gynaecol 1996; 103(12): 1217–21.

94. Suk Wai Ngai, Yik Ming Chan, Pak Chung Ho. Vaginal misoprostol as medical treatment for first trimester spontaneous miscarriage. Hum Reprod 2001; 16:1493–6.

95. Blohm F, Fridén BE, Milsom I, Platz-Christensen JJ, Nielsen S. A randomized double blind trial comparing misoprostol or placebo for the expectant management of early miscarriage. Br J Obstet Gynaecol 2005; 112(8):1090–5.

96. Bagratee JS, Khullar V, Regan L, Moodley J, Kagoro H. A randomized controlled trial comparing medical and expectant management of first trimester miscarriage. Hum Reprod 2004; 19(2):266–71.

97. Blohm F, Hahlin M, Nielsen S, Milson I. A randomised trial comparing fertility after spontaneous abortion managed either by surgical evacuation or expectancy. Lancet 1997; 347:995.

98. Nielsen S, Plats-Christensen JJ. Submitted for publication, 2006.

99. Blohm F, Hahlin M, Nielsen S, Milson I. A randomised trial comparing fertility after spontaneous abortion managed either by surgical evacuation or expectancy. Research letter. Lancet 1997; 347:995.

100. Nielsen S, Hahlin M, Moller A, Granberg S. Bereavement, grieving and psychological morbidity after first trimester spontaneous abortion: comparing expectant management with surgical evacuation. Hum Reprod 1996; 11(8):1767–70.

101. Wieringa-De Waard M, Hartman EE, et al. Expectant management versus surgical evacuation in first trimester miscarriage: health-related quality of life in randomized and non-randomized patients. Hum Reprod 2002; 17(6):1638–42.

6

Medical and surgical management of miscarriage

Johanna Trinder

INTRODUCTION

Traditionally surgical curettage has been performed following the diagnosis of miscarriage, on the assumption that this prevents haemorrhage and decreases the risk of subsequent gynaecological infection. Medical management of miscarriage has been increasingly used as an alternative to surgical management for the past 10 years. Treatment regimens include the use of the antiprogesterone, mifepristone and a prostaglandin analogue, the most commonly used of which is misoprostol (15-deoxy,16-hydroxy,16-methyl analogue of prostaglandin E1). The aim of this chapter is to review the evidence for both medical and surgical management and consider the risks, benefits and practicability of these management options.

MEDICAL MANAGEMENT

Medical management of first trimester miscarriage was considered as an option following the success of medical management for first-trimester therapeutic abortion. Treatment regimens for abortion included initial administration of the antiprogesterone mifepristone, followed 48 hours later by misoprostol. Mifepristone is thought to potentiate the effects of prostaglandins and has been shown to increase the efficacy of misoprostol in the management of therapeutic abortion.[1] Similar regimens gave very high success rates in the management of early fetal demise.[2] However, failing pregnancies are associated with decreased progesterone levels, therefore the necessity for a progesterone antagonist is less clear. It is therefore not surprising that the use of mifepristone in addition to misoprostol has subsequently not been shown to increase the success rate of misoprostol alone in the management of early fetal demise or incomplete miscarriage.[3–5]

Misoprostol is absorbed through mucous membranes and can be administered orally, vaginally, sublingually or rectally. Misoprostol administered via the vaginal route has a greater bioavailability than the oral route. It results in a lower peak concentration, but a longer sustained plasma level.[6] In first-trimester therapeutic abortion, administration via the vaginal route has been shown to be more effective with fewer gastrointestinal side effects.[1] Researchers had suggested that moistening the tablets prior to vaginal administration may benefit absorption,[7] but this has not been shown to be to any advantage in a randomized controlled trial of medical management of miscarriage.[8]

Seven randomized controlled trials of medical (misoprostol) versus surgical management have been published to date.[4,5,9–13] One trial used a partial randomization.[10] Success rates as low as 13%[9] and as high as 93%[12] have been reported in small trials. However, total success was achieved in 50% of women in the largest of these trials, with a sample size of 635 women.[11]

The differences in the success rates of these trials can be attributed to the type of miscarriage treated (whether incomplete or early fetal demise) and dose and route of administration of misoprostol. However, the most important difference in terms of clinical impact, is whether the trials were conducted in an inpatient or outpatient setting (Figure 6.1). The success rates therefore need to be looked at in more detail if we are to understand their significance.

Table 6.1. Suggested regimen for inpatient medical management of early fetal demise
• Admit at time convenient for patient/unit
• Obtain consent for procedure (good practice) Risks – haemorrhage, failure of complete evacuation, infection
• Administer 800 mg vaginal misoprostol
• Thereafter administer oral 400 mg misoprostol at 3 hourly intervals (maximum four oral doses)
• Offer analgesia (oral or parenterally as required). Antiemetics may also be necessary
• Anticipate passage of products of conception in an average of 8 hours (range 2–15 hrs)
• If excessive haemorrhage, remove products of conception from cervical os with sponge forceps
• Examine POC to ensure sac present and send for histological examination
• Administer Anti-D 250 IU if Rhesus negative
• If POC passed and bleeding has subsided – patient may be discharged
• If failure of passage of RPOC; offer repeat course after 12 hours, surgical curettage, allow home and await spontaneous passage of products
• Ask patient to return if bleeding is still present after 2 weeks or if symptoms of infection

Inpatient medical management

In the largest trial, 635 women were randomized to inpatient medical management (4-hourly oral 400 mg misoprostol; three doses, with surgical management the next day if no tissue was passed) or surgical management. A medical success rate of 50% was reported. The average duration of hospital stay was 2.18 days for medical management and 1.78 days for surgical management.[11]

A smaller trial reported a success rate of 82% following the administration of a single vaginal dose of 800 mg misoprostol. Eight to ten hours were allowed for completion of miscarriage. This time period was similar to the average time period (14 hours) from diagnosis to surgical management in the control group.[4]

These trials of inpatient medical management indicate that with an appropriate misoprostol regimen, success, in a similar time span to that required for surgical management, can be attained. A suggested protocol for the inpatient medical management of early fetal demise is detailed in Table 6.1.

Outpatient medical management

Outpatient use of misoprostol compared to surgical management has been evaluated in three trials.[5,12,13]

An efficacy of 60% after 72 hours following the vaginal administration of 800 mg of misoprostol (repeated after 24 hours and 48 hours) has been reported in the management of early fetal demise.[13] The mean time to the expulsion of products was 12.6 hours. Using smaller doses of misoprostol (400 mg then 200 mg 2 hours later), but allowing a longer time period (8 days) for the miscarriage to complete increases the success rates in early fetal demise to 72% (96% surgical).[5]

Allowing a longer time period to complete miscarriage (10 days) whilst utilizing small, repeated doses of misoprostol (200 mg qds for 5 days) results in rates of medical evacuation comparable to those obtained surgically (93% vs 100%), in cases of incomplete miscarriage.[12]

These trials confirm that medical management can be successful in managing miscarriage. It is perhaps more important in practical terms to compare outpatient medical management to expectant management, as these are the options that a woman wanting to avoid surgery will face. Medical and expectant management have been compared in four trials.[3,17–19]

In the first trial of outpatient medical management of early fetal demise, no significant difference was found after 5 days following treatment with a 400 mg oral misoprostol or expectant management (82% vs. 76%).[3]

In a subsequent randomized controlled trial of early fetal demise and incomplete miscarriage, medical management (400 mg misoprostol on days 1, 3, 5) resulted in a complete miscarriage rate of 83% versus 48% ($P < 0.05$) in the expectant group after 14 days.[17]

Two of the trials were double-blind, placebo-controlled trials. Management of early fetal demise (without vaginal bleeding) has been shown to be successful in 80% (20/25) of cases following misoprostol (vaginal administration of up to two doses of 800 mg misoprostol 24 hours apart), compared to 4/25 (16%) receiving placebo ($P < 0.001$) (surgical management was offered after 48 hours if there was no response to the medication).[14] Similar results were also obtained in the medical management of early fetal demise (up to two doses of 600 mg vaginal misoprostol 24 hours apart). Medical management was successful in 87% of women with early fetal demise, compared to 29% of women receiving placebo, following assessment at 7 days.[18] Three-quarters of the women receiving misoprostol were successful within 48 hours (i.e. similar results to Wood et al.[14]). In the same trial there was no significant added benefit for misoprostol over placebo (100% misoprostol vs 86% placebo) in the management of incomplete miscarriage, although the numbers were small. A suggested protocol for the outpatient medical management of early fetal demise is described in Table 6.2.

Table 6.2. Suggested regimen for outpatient medical management of early fetal demise
• Obtain consent for procedure (good practice) Risks – haemorrhage, failure of complete evacuation, infection, failure of diagnosis of gestational trophoblastic disease

• Administer 800 mg vaginal misoprostol and discharge
  – Assuming patient has transport and constant companion
  – If no transport/companion, suggest patient inserts misoprostol at home

• Provide patient with a further 800 mg misoprostol to administer vaginally after 24 hours
  – Suggest insert with tampon, then remove tampon
  – Second dose may be taken orally, but potentially more nausea, vomiting and diarrhoea and is probably less efficacious
  – If misoprostol is to be taken orally, suggest two doses of 400 mg, 3 hours apart

• Patient must be provided with 24-hour emergency contact number and there must be provision for rapid admission if necessary
• Administer Anti-D 250 IU if Rhesus negative (within 72 hours)
• Patient must have access to analgesia (codeine and paracetamol)

• Patient must have written information explaining amount of bleeding to expect
  – Expect more bleeding than with a period
  – Expect passage of clots (may be large)
  – Expect passage of tissue

• Collection of tissue for histological examination is unpleasant, but should be recommended if possible
• Anticipate passage of products of conception within 48 hours in over 80% of women. If no products passed by 7 days offer surgical curettage. Repeat medication could be offered, but no data are available
• Ask patient to return after 2 weeks for transvaginal ultrasound scan and urinary hCG   – If hCG is negative and the woman is symptom free, then repeat a TVS is unnecessary

ROUTE OF ADMINISTRATION OF MISOPROSTOL – ORAL OR VAGINAL?

Single-dose vaginal misoprostol (800 mg) has been shown to be more effective (88% vs 25%)

than oral misoprostol (400 mg) in the management of early fetal demise.[19] This suggests that larger doses of misoprostol given by the vaginal route are more likely to result in successful evacuation. However, when equal doses have been compared in randomized controlled trials, there was no difference in the efficacy of the 800 mg misoprostol administered vaginally or orally (92% vs 89%).[20,21]. However the mean time to expulsion was significantly longer in the oral group[21] and the incidence of diarrhoea was less in the vaginally administered group (14% vs 65%).[20]

The use of a 600 mg single dose of vaginal misoprostol seems to be as effective as three 400 mg oral doses in the management of incomplete miscarriage, with significantly less diarrhoea reported in the vaginally administered group.[22]

Sublingual misoprostol has also been compared to vaginal misoprostol in a randomized controlled trial.[23] Three doses of 600 mg misoprostol were administered at 3-hourly intervals. There was no difference in the efficacy (87.5% vs 95%), but the incidence of diarrhoea was significantly higher in the sublingual (70%) than the vaginal preparation (27.5%) (P <0.005).

Therefore despite the increased bioavailability, there does not seem to be a benefit in efficacy of using the vaginal route over the oral route of administration of misoprostol. The benefit of the vaginal route however may be in the reduced incidence of gastrointestinal side effects and possible shorter administration–expulsion time.

COMPLICATIONS OF MEDICAL MANAGEMENT

Infection

Most published trials are underpowered to detect the infection rate following medical management. The MIST trial[24] (Miscarriage Treatment Trial) reported an infection rate of 2% at 14 days (3% at 8 weeks) based on clinical assessment parameters. The rate of infection was similar to that found in the expectant and surgical groups. A similar infection rate of 3% was reported in a retrospective observational study[25] and in randomized controlled trials.[5,11,12]

Gastrointestinal side effects

Up to 24% of women complain of nausea and 48% of diarrhoea following misoprostol administration (400 mg oral, every 4 hours), compared to 8% and 1% of women receiving surgical management.[11] A meta-analysis of various doses and routes of administration of misoprostol indicates a rate of nausea of 23% and diarrhoea of 18%.[26] Gastrointestinal side effects appear to be less severe if misoprostol is administered via the vaginal rather than the oral or sublingual route.[1,22,23]

Interestingly, the incidence of nausea, vomiting and diarrhoea following 600 mg vaginally administered misoprostol has been recently found to be no different to those receiving vaginally administered placebo (32%, 14% and 21% respectively).[18] More importantly, the incidence of these gastrointestinal complications does not seem to be severe enough to dissuade women from accepting medical management. In a large randomized controlled trial, only 1% of women were unable to continue with misoprostol due to these side effects.[11]

Bleeding

The number of days of vaginal bleeding following medical management is reported to be around 7–15.[5,17] Compared to expectant management, the duration of bleeding is similar, around 11 days.[18]

The risk of heavy bleeding requiring emergency evacuation has been reported at 5%, with a significantly higher risk if the woman has been pre-treated with mifepristone (11% vs 1%, P <0.05).[5] Heavy bleeding requiring blood transfusion may occur in 1% of women pretreated with mifepristone (MIST trial).

Pain

Bagratee et al. found no difference in pain score and analgesia use in the outpatient management of miscarriage with vaginal misoprosostol compared to placebo.[18]

MEDICAL MANAGEMENT IN PRACTICE

Inpatient medical management can be difficult to organize. It is dependent on the availability of an inpatient bed, preferably in a side room to allow some degree of privacy. As both of these resources are relatively scarce, this can be hard to achieve.

The alternative management option would be medical management in an outpatient setting. This appears to be successful and acceptable to women.[18] In terms of management of incomplete miscarriage, there appears to be little increased efficacy over expectant management and therefore managing these women medically may lead to unnecessarily increased rates of gastrointestinal side effects.[3]

The real advantage of medical management is in the outpatient management of early fetal demise, where the success rates vastly supersede those of expectant management. There appears to be no difference in the success rates of medical management with regard to gestation sac size or crown–rump length.[5] Unlike expectant management, the absence of vaginal bleeding does not decrease the success rates.[18]

Although still not absolutely clear, the evidence suggests optimal management is with vaginally administered misoprostol, presumably ensuring effective blood levels with minimal side effects. In terms of practicability it would be beneficial perhaps to give one vaginal dose of misoprostol in the early pregnancy clinic, to ensure optimal bioavailability. Then either prescribe oral, lower misoprostol doses to be administered at home or a further dose of vaginal misoprostol (which has been shown to be successfully self-inserted).[21,27]

As for expectant management, women need to be informed in no uncertain terms of the amount of bleeding and pain that they are likely to experience and the diarrhoea and vomiting that they may expect as side effects of misoprostol. If the patient is not likely to be compliant then a conservative management approach is not a safe option. If medical management fails and surgical curettage is carried out, it appears that there may be less surgery-related complications, probably due to the softening effect on the cervix allowing easier instrumentation of the uterine cavity.[26]

Outpatient medical management should however only be practiced in units which have the facility for 24-hour contact and the option to review and potentially admit patients who experience excessive pain and/or haemorrhage.

EXCLUSIONS TO MEDICAL MANAGEMENT

Women should not be offered medical management if there are signs or symptoms of infection or severe haemorrhage. Misoprostol can cause vascular dilatation and therefore hypotension, therefore it should be used with caution (i.e. certainly not as an outpatient) in women with cardiac disease (especially mitral stenosis). It should also be avoided in women with glaucoma.

SURGICAL MANAGEMENT OF MISCARRIAGE

Surgical management includes dilatation and curettage (D&C, using a sharp metal curette) and suction curettage (using a metal or more commonly plastic cannula and a vacuum, via an electric or foot-pump, or with a hand-held manual vacuum device). D&C has been replaced by suction curettage as the usual surgical technique for early fetal demise, but is still used for the management of incomplete miscarriage.[28] Suction curettage for incomplete miscarriage has however been shown to be associated with less blood loss and pain than sharp curettage.[29]

In a meta-analysis of women undergoing surgical curettage as the control group in RCTs of expectant and medical management of pregnancy failure, the rate of complete evacuation was 97%.[26] This makes it the most efficacious option in the management of miscarriage.

Surgical curettage, however, is not without complications. These include: cervical damage; perforation; intra-abdominal trauma; intrauterine adhesions; haemorrhage; and the potential to introduce infection as a result of uterine instrumentation. There are also the risks associated with a general anaesthetic. Some practical points relating to surgical management are detailed in Table 6.3.

Table 6.3. Surgical curettage

- Cervical/urethral swab for *Chlamydia* (or urinary PCR if heavy bleeding)
- Misoprostol vaginal 400 mg 2 hours before procedure
- Anaesthesia
  - General
  - Spinal
  - Local (paracervical ± sedation)
- Dilatation of cervical canal (to maximum of Hegar 12)
- Vacuum aspiration using Karmen or Corey curette
- Check cavity is empty using curette
- Ensure bleeding has subsided
- Analgesia
- Send all tissue obtained for histological analysis
- 250 IU anti-D if Rhesus negative

COMPLICATIONS OF SURGICAL MANAGEMENT

Risks of cervical or uterine damage

The risk of cervical tears, uterine perforation and Asherman's syndrome, based on meta-analyses, seems to be in the order of 0.79% to 1.9%.[26]

Risks of haemorrhage

The risk of haemorrhage following suction curettage is in the order of 0.24 to 3.2%.[26]

Risk of infection

Infection rates of 3–4% for surgical curettage have been found in larger trials and a meta-analysis of pooled data[11,26] and confirmed by the MIST trial.

The impact of infection on long-term fertility is particularly important when the organism in question is either *Chlamydia* or gonorrhoea. The rate of postoperative infection with *Chlamydia* and/or gonorrhoea in the USA for women undergoing suction curettage for incomplete miscarriage is reported to be 6%.[30] This rate is unchanged by the use of doxycycline prophy-

laxis, although this trial may have been under-powered to detect a difference. The routine use of antibiotic prophylaxis in reducing the incidence of pelvic infection has been clearly demonstrated in induced abortion (see RCOG National Evidence-based Guideline No 7). Until further research is published, the RCOG recommends that all at-risk women undergoing surgical evacuation continue to be screened for *Chlamydia trachomatis*.[31] This particularly applies to women under the age of 25.[28]

Vaginal bleeding

The number of days reported with vaginal bleeding following surgical management ranges between 3 days[5] and 9 days.[32]

Manual vacuum aspiration

Despite the superior success rate, up to 75% of women will choose expectant as an alternative to surgical management.[33] This decision, in some women is in order to avoid an 'operation' with its inherent risks.[34] It is usual practice in the UK to manage miscarriage by performing electric suction curettage under general anaesthetic.[27] In the developing world, however, manual vacuum aspiration (MVA) performed under local anaesthetic is widely used. In the UK, there is increasing experience using this technique in the management of early first-trimester termination. Manual vacuum aspiration appears to be as safe as electric suction curettage for therapeutic abortions up to 10 weeks' gestation.[35] This technique has been recently evaluated for the management of incomplete miscarriage and early fetal demise, using systemic analgesia (intravenous alfentanil and midazolam) and patient-controlled analgesia (alfentanil and propofol).[36] Although experience with miscarriage is limited, MVA may prove to be acceptable to women requesting early resolution of their miscarriage, but wanting to avoid general anaesthesia. It should be possible to develop this technique to manage miscarriage in a modified outpatient setting.

MISOPROSTOL FOR CERVICAL RIPENING PRIOR TO SUCTION CURETTAGE

Misoprostol can be used for cervical ripening; namely softening, effacement and gradual dilatation of the cervical os. This process makes gaining access to the uterine cavity technically easier and has been shown to reduce the incidence of cervical lacerations and uterine perforation at the time of first-trimester therapeutic abortion. It appears that the most suitable dose is 400 mg of vaginal misoprostol, preferably inserted 3–4 hours before suction curettage.[37]

Rh IMMUNIZATION

There is evidence that significant fetomaternal haemorrhage can occur after curettage to remove products of conception but does not occur after complete spontaneous miscarriage. It is difficult to ascertain the risk incurred following medical management. The RCOG have therefore recommended that anti-D should be given to all non-sensitized Rh-negative women who miscarry after 12 weeks, whether complete or incomplete and to those who miscarry below 12 weeks when the uterus is evacuated[38] (either surgically or medically[28]).

HISTOLOGICAL EXAMINATION

The Royal College of Obstetricians and Gynaecologists has recommended that all women should have pregnancy tissue sent for histological examination.[28] There is evidence that this does not happen in 30% of cases treated in hospital (i.e. surgical and medical management).[39] This recommendation was derived from the consensus opinion of an expert group.[31] The purpose of the recommendation was to safeguard against the missed diagnosis of ectopic pregnancy and trophoblastic disease. There are no data on the frequency of histological examination in women who undergo expectant management at home, but for outpatient medical management, it is probably unrealistic to expect women to miscarry at home, collect tissue and return it to the early pregnancy clinic, although currently this should be advised.

PSYCHOLOGICAL EFFECTS OF MEDICAL VERSUS SURGICAL MANAGEMENT

In randomized controlled trials to compare the psychological impact of surgical with medical management, no difference has been observed in psychological outcomes.[10,40] In measuring client satisfaction overall, significantly more women would choose to undergo surgical management, rather than medical management if they suffered a further miscarriage.[10] However, significantly more women who experience successful evacuation of the uterus with misoprostol would choose the same mode of treatment if they were able to choose again, but not surprisingly women for whom medical treatment failed to evacuate the uterus and subsequent surgical evacuation was required are significantly less satisfied with the treatment.[40]

SUMMARY

There are increasingly more objective data from randomized controlled trials (RCTs) (Table 6.4) assessing which management option is best for managing miscarriage with respect to complete emptying of the uterine cavity and subsequent uterine infection and other complications. No published trial to date has assessed all three possible options in one trial. RCTs have largely been unsuccessful in recruiting large numbers of women as it is difficult to recruit women at such an emotional time, and as many as eight out of nine women express a definite preference for treatment and decline randomization.[41]

Evidence from pooling data from randomized controlled trials of expectant vs. surgical, expectant vs. medical and medical vs. surgical management of miscarriage suggests that the infection rates are not significantly different and are reassuringly low. This is despite the fact that neither screening for infection, nor prophylactic antibiotics were used in many of the trials. Table 6.4 outlines the data relating to randomized trials of medical management. These data should be reassuring to those who have previously raised concern about the lack of evidence available for non-surgical treatment of miscarriage.[42,43]

Table 6.4. Randomised controlled trials of medical management

Authors	Year	Miscarriage type	Inclusion criteria	Treatment regimen	Success Expectant	Medical	Surgical	P value
Inpatient								
de Jonge[9]	1995	Incomplete	clinical assessment	400 mg oral misoprostol		3/23 (13%)	26/27 (96%)	<0.00001
Herabutya[46]	1996	EFD	USS but criteria not stated	200 mg vaginal misoprostol	6/42 (17%)	35/42 (83%)		<0.0001
Hinshaw[10] (partial randomization)	1997	EFD	Not stated	400/600/400 mg oral mifepristone 2 h apart		172/186 (93%)	247/251(98%)	=0.004
		Incomplete	Not stated	400/200 mg oral misoprostol 2 h apart		57/57 (100%)	27/27 (100%)	
Chung[11]	1999	EFD & incomplete		3 × 400 µg oral misoprostol at 3 hour intervals		159/321 (50%)	299/314 (95%)	
Demetroulis[4]	2001	EFD & incomplete	ET>15 mm RCT/RCOG	800 mg vaginal misoprostol		33/40 (82%)	40/40 (100%)	=0.005
Outpatient								
Nielsen[3]	1999	EFD & incomplete	ET>15 mm & RCR/RCOG	400 mg misoprostol	47/62 (76%)	49/60 (82%)		
Ngai[47]	2001	EFD	RCOG/RCR	3 × 400 mg vaginal misoprostol days 1, 3, 5	14/29 (48%)	25/30 (83%)		<0.05
Sahin[12]	2001	Incomplete	ET<50 mm	200 mg vaginal misoprostol then 200 mg qds po for 5 days		37/40 (93)%	40/40 (100%)	
Muffley[13]	2002	EFD	CRL >5 mm	800 mg misoprostol repeated if necessary 24, 48 hours		15/25 (60%)	25/25 (100%)	
Wood[14]	2002	EFD	MSD 16 mm	800 mg vaginal misoprostol	4/25 (16%)	20/25 (80%)		RR 0.20 (0.08, 0.50) <0.001
Bagratee[18]	2004	EFD incomplete	RCOG/RCR ET>15	600 mg vaginal misorostol repeated if necessary after 24 hours	11/38 (29%) 12/14 (86%)	39/45 (87%) 7/7 (100%)		OR 15.96 95%CI (5.26–48.37)
Gronlund[5]	2002	EFD	CRL 6–20 mm MSD >15mm	400/200 mg vaginal misoprostol 2 h apart		92/127 (72%)	47/49 (96%)	

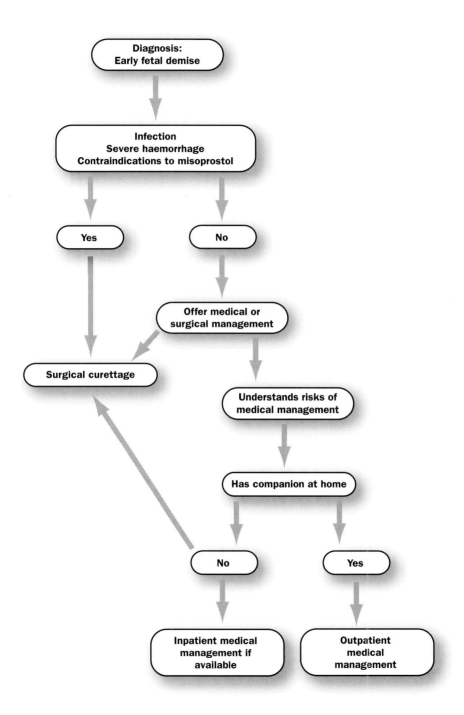

Figure 6.1 Decision tree for management of early fetal demise

There is a wide variation in the success rates reported by individual studies and trials of medical management. It is difficult to directly compare these success rates, as researchers have used different entry criteria, treatment regimens and end-points.

Women are increasingly offered a choice of treatment for management of their miscarriage. The unplanned admission rates in women randomized to expectant management confirms the RCOG advice that medical management should only be offered in units where patients have access to 24-hour telephone advice and immediate admission can be arranged.[28] Medical management does not offer significant success over expectant management when used to treat incomplete miscarriage, but offers a non-surgical alternative management in early fetal demise. Inpatient medical management of early fetal demise may initially seem attractive, but success rates are higher if a longer time period for products of conception to pass is allowed and the increased time spent in hospital could be seen as unattractive to women and care providers alike. A published economic analysis of medical management estimates a similar cost to surgical management, but this is based on an optimistic success rate in excess of 90% and a usual inpatient stay of 6–8 hours.[44]

A more practical approach is to use misoprostol in an outpatient setting. Randomized trials have shown that this is possible with success rates of 87% for early fetal demise.[18] It appears that the vaginal route may be optimal, at least for the initial dose. Further work needs to be undertaken to identify the optimal efficacious dose that can be balanced against low incidence of side effects and is suitable for self-administration.

Success rates if anything will be higher than randomized controlled trials suggest, as women who choose, rather than are randomized to a treatment option are likely to be more motivated to follow their chosen treatment to completion.[45]

CONCLUSION

For women with incomplete miscarriage, expectant management should be actively encouraged, as at least 75% of women will be successful with no increased risk of infection. Ideally medical or surgical management should be offered to women with a diagnosis of early fetal and embryonic demise. Medical management is at least 80% successful in the outpatient setting for management of early fetal demise. Surgical curettage still offers the greatest success rate (97%), the least risk of requiring unplanned admission and the least duration of bleeding. It should therefore continue to be offered as a management option, particularly to those women with early fetal demise who do not wish to undergo the uncertainty, nor the procedure associated with therapeutic management.

CASE REPORT 1

Mrs PB, G5P4, age 36, attends the Early Pregnancy Unit complaining of vaginal bleeding at 8 weeks' gestation. Transvaginal ultrasound reveals a fetus of 7 mm CRL with no visible heart activity. Early fetal demise is diagnosed. Expectant, medical or surgical management are offered. Mrs B chooses surgical management as she has four young children at home and is unable to accept the uncertainty of expectant or medical management. She is booked for evacuation of retained products (ERPC) the following day as a day-case procedure. The procedure is uneventful and Mrs B is discharged 2 hours postoperatively. The products are sent for histological examination. She continues to bleed vaginally for a further 5 days. No follow-up is arranged. Mrs B is relieved that it is all over so quickly and she can return to 'normal'.

CASE REPORT 2

Miss LA, G1P0, age 23, attends the Early Pregnancy Unit complaining of brown vaginal discharge at 9 weeks' gestation. Transvaginal ultrasound scan reveals an empty gestation sac with a mean diameter of 25 mm. Early fetal demise is diagnosed and Miss LA is offered expectant, medical or surgical management. She chooses medical management as she feels that a success rate of over 80% is worth trying, especially as it avoids hospitalization and a general anaesthetic. She is given 800 mg of vaginal misoprostol and sent home. Her mother is able to stay with her. She experiences some cramps a few hours after the misoprostol is given, but no products are passed. She self-administers a further 800 mg of misoprostol 24 hours later. A few hours after this second dose, vaginal bleeding is increased and severe pelvic cramps occur. She takes some co-dydramol for the pain. One hour later she passes clots and a lump of 'jelly'-like substance. She disposes of the tissue down the lavatory. The pain subsides, the bleeding is, however, 'like a period'. The vaginal bleeding reduces over the next 5 days and by 8 days, stops.

Miss LA returns to the early pregnancy unit after 2 weeks. Urinary hCG is negative and transvaginal ultrasound shows an empty uterus. Miss LA says that the experience was 'awful', but in her view, preferable to having to be admitted to hospital and have a general anaesthetic.

PRACTICAL POINTS

Comparison of the medical and surgical management of miscarriage

	Medical	Surgical
Advantages	Avoids anaesthetic Can be undertaken at home	Booked procedure Completed quickly
Disadvantages	Can be unpleasant Time period to completion uncertain	Requires anaesthetic Usually requires hospital admission
Success	More than 80%	97%
Time required	Mostly within 48 hours	Admission for 4–8 hours
Complications	Haemorrhage Infection Emergency admission	Haemorrhage Perforation/cervical trauma Infection
Side effects	Pain Nausea Vomiting	Pain Nausea Vomiting
Bleeding	12 days	9 days
Psychological effects	No difference	No difference
Patient satisfaction	Higher if successful Less if unsuccessful	High

---

REFERENCES

1. Kulier R, Gulmezoglu A, Hofmeyr G, Cheng L, Campana A. Medical methods for first trimester abortion. Cochrane Database, 2004; Syst Rev 2 [CD002855].
2. el Refaey H, Hinshaw K, Henshaw R, Smith N, Templeton A. Medical management of missed abortion and anembryonic pregnancy. BMJ 1992; 305:1399.
3. Nielsen S, Hahlin M, Platz-Christensen J. Randomised trial comparing expectant with medical management for first trimester miscarriages. Br J Obstet Gynaecol 1999; 106(8):804–7.
4. Demetroulis C, Saridogan E, Kunde D, Naftalin A. A prospective randomised control trial comparing medical and surgical treatment for early pregnancy failure. Hum Reprod 2001; 16(2):365–9.
5. Gronlund A, Gronlund L, Clevin L, et al. Management of missed abortion: comparison of medical treatment

with either mifepristone + misoprostol or misoprostol alone with surgical evacuation. A multi-center trial in Copenhagen county, Denmark. Acta Obstet Gynecol Scand 2002; 81(11):1060–5.

6. Zieman M, Fong S, Benowitz N, Banskter D, Darney P. Absorption kinetics of misoprostol with oral or vaginal administration. Obstet Gynecol 1997; 90(1):88–92.

7. Zalanyi S. Vaginal misoprostol alone is effective in the treatment of missed abortion. Br J Obstet Gynaecol 1998; 105(9):1026–8.

8. Miles J, Creinin MD, Barnhart K, et al. A randomized trial of saline-moistened misoprostol versus dry misoprostol for first-trimester pregnancy failure. Am J Obstet Gynecol 2004; 190(2)389–94.

9. de Jonge ET, Makin JD, Manefeldt E, De Wet GH, Pattinson RC. Randomised clinical trial of medical evacuation and surgical curettage for incomplete miscarriage. BMJ 1995; 311(7006):662.

10. Hinshaw K. Medical management of miscarriage. In: Grudzinskas JG, O'Brien P, eds. Problems in early pregnancy: Advances in diagnosis and management. London: Royal College of Obstetricians and Gynaecologists, 1997: 284–93.

11. Chung TK, Lee DT, Cheung LP, Haines CJ, Chang AM. Spontaneous abortion: a randomized, controlled trial comparing surgical evacuation with conservative management using misoprostol. Fertil Steril 1999; 71(6):1054–9.

12. Sahin HG, Sahin HA, Kocer M. Randomized outpatient clinical trial of medical evacuation and surgical curettage in incomplete miscarriage. Eur J Contracept Reprod Health Care 2001; 6(3):141–4.

13. Muffley PE, Stitely ML, Gherman RB. Early intrauterine pregnancy failure: a randomized trial of medical versus surgical treatment. Am J Obstet Gynecol 2002; 00:321–5.

14. Wood SL, Brain PH. Medical management of missed abortion: a randomised controlled trial. Obstet Gynaecol 2002; 99(4):563–6.

15. Creinin MD, Harwood B, Guido R. Medical management of missed abortion: a randomised controlled trial. Obstet Gynaecol 2002; 100(2):382–3.

16. Kovavisarach E, Sathapanachai U. Intravaginal 400 microg misoprostol for pregnancy termination in cases of blighted ovum: a randomised controlled trial. NZ J Obstet Gynaecol 2002; 42(2):161–3.

17. Ngai SW, Chan YM, Tang OS, Ho PC. Vaginal misoprostol as medical treatment for first trimester spontaneous miscarriage. Hum Reprod 2001; 16AB(7):1493–6.

18. Bagratee J, Khullar V, Regan L, Moodley J, Kagoro H. A randomized controlled trial comparing medical and expectant management of first trimester miscarriage. Hum Reprod 2004; 19(2):266–71.

19. Creinin MD, Moyer R, Guido R. Misoprostol for medical evacuation of early pregnancy failure. Obstet Gynecol 1997; 89:768–72.

20. Pang MW, Lee TS, Chung TK. Incomplete miscarriage: a randomized controlled trial comparing oral with vaginal misoprostol for medical evacuation. Hum Reprod 2001; 16(11):2283–7.

21. Ngoc N, Blum J, Westheimer E, Quan T, Winikoff B. Medical treatment of missed abortion using misoprostol. Int J Gynaecol Obstet 2004; 87:138–142.

22. Phupong V, Taneepanichskul S, Kriengsinyot R, et al. Comparative study between single dose 600 microgrammes and repeated dose of oral misoprostol for treatment of incomplete abortion. Contraception 2004; 70(4):307–11.

23. Tang OS, Lau WN, Ng EH, Lee SW, Ho PC. A prospective randomized study to compare the use of repeated doses of vaginal with sublingual misoprostol in the management of first trimester silent miscarriages. Hum Reprod 2003; 18(1):176–81.

24. Trinder J, Brocklehurst P, Porter R, et al. Management of miscarriage: expectant, medical, or surgical? Results of randomised controlled trial (miscarriage treatment (MIST) trial). BMJ 2006; 332:235–8.

25. Greenland H, Ogunbiyi I, Bugg G, Tasker M. Medical treatment of miscarriage in a district general hospital is safe and effective up to 12 weeks' gestation. Curr Med Res Opin 2005; 00(0):699–701.

26. Graziosi G, Mol B, Ankum W, Bruinse H.. Management of early pregnancy loss. Int J Gynaecol Obstet 2004; 86(3):337–46.

27. Schaff EA, Fielding SL, Westhoff C, et al. Vaginal misoprostol administered 1, 2, or or 3 days after mifepristone for early medical abortion: A randomized trial. JAMA 2000; 284(15):1948–53.

28. Hinshaw K, Fernandez H. The management of early pregnacy loss. Clinical Green Top Guidelines. Royal College Obstetricians and Gynaecologists, 2002

29. Forna F, Gulmezoglu A. Surgical procedures to evacuate incomplete abortion. The Cochrane Database of Systemic Reviews [1. Art. No.: CD001993. DOI: 10.1002/14651858.CD001993]. 2001.

30. Prieto J, Eriksen N, Blanco J. A randomized trial of prophylactic doxycycline for curettage in incomplete abortion. Obstet Gynecol 1995; 85(5):692–6.

31. RCOG Study Group. Recommendations from the 33rd RCOG study group. In: Grudzinskas JG, O'Brien P, eds. Problems in early pregnancy: advances in diagnosis and management. London: RCOG Press, 1997: 327–31

32. Nielsen S, Hahlin M. Expectant management of first-trimester spontaneous abortion. Lancet 1995; 345:84–6.

33. Luise C, Jermy K, Collins WP, Bourne TH. Expectant management of incomplete, spontaneous first-

trimester miscarriage: outcome according to initial ultrasound criteria and value of follow-up visits. Ultrasound Obstet Gynecol 2002; 19:580–2.

34. Ogden J, Maker C. Expectant or surgical management of miscarriage: a qualitative study. BJOG 2004; iii:463–7.

35. Goldberg AB, Dean G, Kang MS, Youssof S, Darney PD. Manual versus electric vacuum aspiration for early first-trimester abortion: a controlled study of complication rates. Obstet Gynecol 2004; 103(1):101–7.

36. Gazvani R, Honey E, MacLennan F, Templeton A. Manual vacuum aspiration (MVA) in the management of first trimester pregnancy loss. Eur J Obstet Gynecol Reprod Biol 2004; 112:197–200.

37. Goldberg AB, Greenberg MB, Darney PD. Misoprostol and pregnancy. N Engl J Med 2001; 000(0):38–47.

38. Robson S. Use of anti-D immunoglobulin for Rh prophylaxis. RCOG Clinical Green Top Guidelines, 2002.

39. Cameron M, Penny G. Are national recommendations regarding examination and disposal of products of miscarriage being followed? A need for revised guidelines. Hum Reprod 2004; 00:531–5.

40. Lee DT, Cheung LP, Haines CJ, Chan KP, Chung TK. A comparison of the psychologic impact and client satisfaction of surgical treatment with medical treatment of spontaneous abortion: a randomized controlled trial. Am J Obstet Gynecol 2001; 185(4):953–8.

41. Hamilton-Fairley D, Donaghy J. Surgical versus expectant management of first-trimester miscarriage: a prospective observational study. In: Grudzinskas JG, O'Brien P, eds. Problems in early pregnancy: Advances in diagnosis and management. London: RCOG Press, 1997: 277–83.

42. Jurkovic D. Modern management of miscarriage: is there a place for non-surgical treatment? [editorial]. Ultrasound Obstet Gynecol 1998; 11(3):161–3.

43. Cahill DJ. Managing spontaneous first trimester miscarriage. BMJ 1991; 322:1315–16.

44. Hughes J, Ryan M, Hinshaw K, et al. The costs of treating miscarriage: a comparison of medical and surgical management. Br J Obstet Gynaecol 1996; 103:1217–21.

45. Brewin T, Thornton H, Bradley C, et al. Patients' preferences and randomised trials. Lancet North Am Ed 1996; 347:1118–19.

46. Herabutya Y, Prasertsawat P. Misoprostol in the management of missed abortion. Int J Gynaecol Obstet 1997; 56(3):263–6.

47. Ngai SW, Chan YM, Tang OS, Ho PC. Vaginal misoprostol as medical treatment for first trimester spontaneous miscarriage. Hum Reprod 2001; 16:1493–6.

EDITORIAL COMMENT

In our view the care given to women suffering from miscarriage has often been very poor. Leaving women bleeding in emergency rooms for hours to be examined by the least experienced gynaecologist available was often normal practice, as was admitting patients pending an ultrasound scan to be performed. This was followed invariably by a curettage procedure at some time later. Fortunately this has changed. The introduction of dedicated early pregnancy units having done much to rectify things.

The major change in the management of miscarriage has been the move away from this being a condition that is seen as requiring a 'surgical solution' to one that can be managed either medically of by simply allowing nature to take its course. It was brave of Sven Neilsen and others to challenge the existing orthodoxy and suggest that it was acceptable to do this. It seems clear now that for incomplete miscarriage, expectant management will succeed in the majority of cases. If there is a gestation sac in the uterus with or without an embryo, then medical management offers advantages. For many women surgery will still be required either because of a medical indication such as bleeding and pain, or because they choose the surgical option. It is important to remember this, as conservative management will not suit all women. The rapid resolution of a highly emotive problem is a positive benefit of surgery. Sometimes we are too keen to push the conservative management approach, both for miscarriage and ectopic pregnancy. Giving women choice in pregnancy means exactly that, and although not necessarily in vogue, surgery will continue to be a mainstay of management for early pregnancy complications.

The anxiety associated with early pregnancy has led to many women having early scans in order to reassure them that all is well. It is of great importance that those performing the scans know what is normal, and it is questionable whether this development is in the interests of the patient. There are few if any data to suggest that screening women in this way is of value. What we do know is that it can be unhelpful. Frequently women are asked to return for repeat scans because either they are classified as having a pregnancy of unknown location or they have a small gestation sac and viability cannot be established. This leads to the possibility of iatrogenic error; diagnosing either miscarriage or ectopic pregnancy inappropriately. It also leads to significant patient anxiety. There is an urgent need to assess the impact of these early scans.

The sensitivities involved in managing early pregnancy loss are obvious. Miscarriage is an inevitable part of reproductive life, but it is hard for couples to see it in that context in a world where individuals expect to control every aspect of their lives. Whatever the technicalities of management, emotional support is a major part of the function of an early pregnancy unit irrespective of how the miscarriage is handled.

7

What do you do when you cannot see a pregnancy? The management of pregnancies of unknown location (PUL)

George Condous

Introduction • What to do? • Mathematical models in the prediction of failing pregnancies of unknown location • Can logistic regression analysis predict the outcome of a pregnancy of unknown location? • The practical application of a mathematical model • New markers in the management of pregnancies of unknown location • Uterine curettage in the management of pregnancies of unknown location • Case report 1 • Case report 2 • Conclusions • Practical points

INTRODUCTION

As we have heard already, the availability of highly sensitive home pregnancy tests and access to walk-in early-pregnancy units (EPUs) has led to an increase in women undergoing early transvaginal ultrasound scans (TVS) to locate, date and confirm the viability of their pregnancy. As more women present at earlier gestations to an EPU, the number classified with a pregnancy of unknown location (PUL) will also increase. We know that the pregnancy site will not be visualized by TVS in 8–31% of women who present to an EPU.[1–9] The prevalence of PULs is determined by the quality of ultrasound scanning.[10] An experienced ultrasonographer will tend to pick up more early intrauterine gestational sacs or adnexal masses compared with an inexperienced one, which in turn will result in a lower prevalence of PULs or non-diagnostic scans for a given EPU.

The acronym PUL is a descriptive term rather than a pathological diagnosis. PULs can be defined as a situation in which there is a positive pregnancy test with no signs of either an intra- or extrauterine pregnancy on TVS. Within the PUL population there are four potential clinical outcomes: a failing PUL, an intrauterine pregnancy (IUP), an ectopic pregnancy or a persisting PUL. The failing PULs (44–69%)[1,3–6] are never visualized using TVS and an indeterminate proportion of these are failing ectopic pregnancies as well as failing intrauterine pregnancies. The persisting PUL group only accounts for 2% of the total PULs.[11] These PULs behave biochemically like ectopic pregnancies and almost certainly represent ultrasonically missed ectopic pregnancies.

WHAT TO DO?

There are some important questions that need to be answered before discussing management. First and foremost, is the diagnosis of a PUL appropriate? Secondly, is the woman clinically stable? And thirdly, has the presence of blood in the pelvis been excluded on the ultrasound scan? Provided that the ultrasound examiner is sufficiently skilled and uses an ultrasound system with acceptable image quality, then the diagnosis is certainly appropriate. If the woman is not clinically stable and/or haemoperitoneum is present on scan, then it is not appropriate to manage such women expectantly. Conversely, if clinically stable and there are no signs of haemoperitoneum on scan then a hands-off, non-interventional approach on an outpatient basis is the most appropriate way forward. This expectant management approach is safe[1-9] as the vast majority of PULs are low-risk PULs and represent failing PULs or very early IUP.[1,11] A 'wait-and-see' approach has been shown to be safe, reduce the need for unnecessary surgical intervention and is not associated with any serious adverse outcomes.[1-9] We have unpublished data at St George's Hospital, London, on more than 1000 consecutive women with a PUL and the overall rate of intervention in the form of a laparoscopy or evacuation of retained products is 8.2%. In this series there were no significant adverse outcomes.

Expectant management with serial biochemical follow up allows the clinician to triage women with a PUL into low-risk and high-risk PULs. Serum levels of hCG and/or progesterone should be taken at presentation and 48 hours later, with the interpretation of the results dictating the subsequent management. It is the calculation of the hCG ratio,[11,12] defined as the hCG at 48 hours divided by the hCG at 0 hours (hCG 48 h/hCG 0 h), that determines the subsequent management. If the serum hCG levels fall by more than 13% in the first 48 h, i.e. the hCG ratio cut-off is <0.87,[12] then these women almost certainly have a failing PUL and should have a repeat serum hCG 1 week later to confirm the diagnosis. Remember a repeat scan in this subgroup of PULs is not necessary as the failing PULs are never seen on follow up scans and represent either complete miscarriages or self-limiting forms of ectopic pregnancy. A serum progesterone of <20 nmol/L at presentation also correlates well with spontaneously resolving PULs.[6] If serum hCG levels increase by more than 66% in 48 h, i.e. an hCG cut-off of >1.66, then this subgroup of women almost certainly have an early IUP and should have a repeat scan 1 week later to confirm the diagnosis. This well-known algorithm is not without its pitfalls, as approximately 13% of ectopic

pregnancies will have an hCG ratio of >1.66.[13] If this is the case, then approximately 1.3% of the total PUL population would behave in this way. Traditionally, women whose hCG ratios do not conform to these cut-offs, i.e. an hCG ratio of >0.87 and <1.66, are called back immediately for a repeat scan and undergo close follow up to exclude an ectopic pregnancy. We have rationalized our management of women with PULs in an attempt to reduce follow up visits. Over the last 12 months we have rescanned this subgroup of PULs with non-conforming hCG ratios at 7 days without any serious adverse outcomes (Figure 7.1).

Traditionally, single variable diagnostic tests have been used in the management of PULs. However, the evaluation of serum hormone levels at defined times in PULs can only be used reliably to predict the immediate viability of a PUL, not its location.[1] The established criteria for the prediction of ectopic pregnancy are based on discriminatory zones for serum hCG and were developed in symptomatic women presenting with abdominal pain and vaginal bleeding.[2,8,14-17] This is a different population to women with an underlying ectopic pregnancy in a PUL population who tend to be clinically stable and relatively asymptomatic. The current criteria for the prediction of ectopic pregnancy therefore do not apply in these cases. Newer more sensitive reproducible models are required for the distinction between ectopic and non-ectopic pregnancies in the PUL population.

In a more recent study in our unit, the diagnostic accuracy of various discriminatory zones (serum hCG of >1000 IU/L, 1500 IU/L and 2000 IU/L) for the prediction of ectopic pregnancy was evaluated.[10] The accuracy of the discriminatory zone for the detection of ectopic pregnancies in this specialist scanning unit was found to be much lower than in non-scanning based units.[10] This is because more relatively early ectopic pregnancies are directly visualized and this group of ectopic pregnancies often have serum hCG levels below any currently used cut-off value for hCG. As the prevalence of ectopic pregnancies in a PUL population increases, so too does the effectiveness of the discriminatory zone as a result of larger ectopic pregnancies not being seen. Hence hCG levels will often be

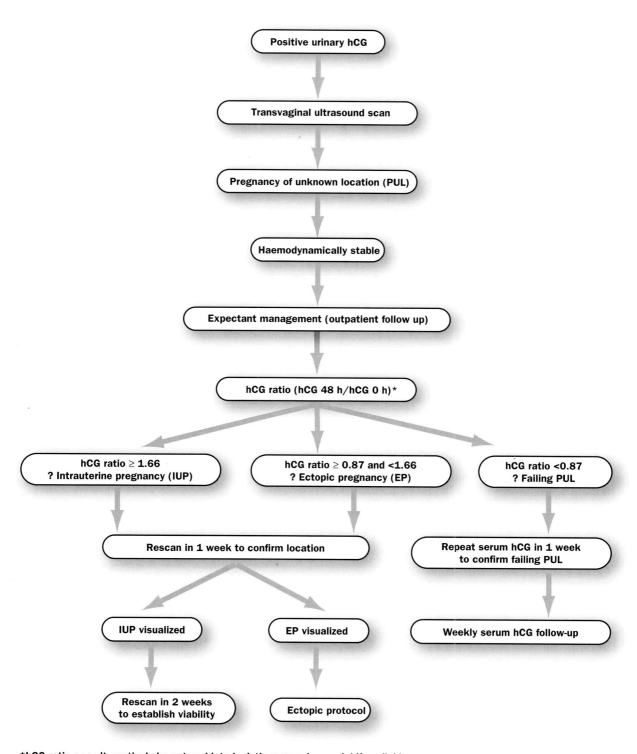

*hCG ratio can alternatively be entered into logistic regression model if available

Figure 7.1 Flow diagram to illustrate a suggested management plan for women with a pregnancy of unknown location.

relatively high. So cut-off values are not without relevance as in some units up to 40% of the PUL population are found to have ectopic pregnancies. In contrast in specialist scanning units most ectopic pregnancies are diagnosed using ultrasound as the primary diagnostic tool, and so they constitute only 8–14%[1,4] of the PUL population. It is our view therefore that using discriminatory zones as a basis to manage these women is not ideal – although we acknowledge that they may still be required when there is a lack of trained ultrasonographers. This lack of test performance has led to the development of mathematical modelling techniques to predict ectopic pregnancies and rationalize follow up in the PUL population.

MATHEMATICAL MODELS IN THE PREDICTION OF FAILING PREGNANCIES OF UNKNOWN LOCATION

Mathematical models have previously been developed to predict the spontaneous resolution of pregnancies in a PUL population. Hahlin et al. developed a model which combined serum progesterone and serial hCG measurements.[3] In their study, the model predicted spontaneous resolution of pregnancy with a sensitivity and specificity of 73% and 97% respectively. In a second approach, the combination of clinical, ultrasonographic and two biochemical parameters were incorporated into a logistic regression model.[4] At the initial visit, the diagnosis of a spontaneously resolving pregnancy was made with a sensitivity and specificity of 92%. In a follow-up study by the same unit, the performance of these mathematical models was no better than a single measurement of serum progesterone of <20 nmol/L for the assessment of women with PULs.[6] Serum progesterone measurements alone can be used to identify spontaneously resolving pregnancies in a PUL population.

CAN LOGISTIC REGRESSION ANALYSIS PREDICT THE OUTCOME OF A PREGNANCY OF UNKNOWN LOCATION?

More recently, our unit has generated and evaluated new logistic regression models from simple demographic and hormonal data to predict the outcome of PULs.[11] The logistic regression model M1, which was based on the hCG ratio, not only predicted the ectopic pregnancy group but also the failing PUL and the IUP groups. The costs of misdiagnosing an ectopic pregnancy are greater than misdiagnosing a failing PUL and an IUP. In this study, we therefore used the weighting for the misclassification of a failing PUL, IUP and ectopic pregnancy: 1, 1 and 4. When the model was weighted to pick up more ectopic pregnancies at the expense of the failing PULs and IUPs, it had a sensitivity of 91.7%, a specificity of 84.2%, a positive likelihood ratio of 5.8, a positive predictive value of 27.5% and a negative predictive value of 99.4% for the prediction of ectopic pregnancies. This model outperformed a discriminatory zone of 1000 IU/L in the same study.

In this study, gestational age and endometrial thickness were found not to be important variables in the development of the logistic regression models. This finding is corroborated in a study by Mol et al. which also reported that gestational age and endometrial thickness were not useful in the diagnosis of ectopic pregnancy.[18]

THE PRACTICAL APPLICATION OF A MATHEMATICAL MODEL

Such mathematical models have been evaluated in the clinical setting in our unit.[19] The logistic regression model, M1, based on the hCG ratio, detected ectopic pregnancies, intrauterine pregnancies and failing PULs with sensitivities of 88.9%, 86.8% and 73.5%, respectively. This model M1 compared favourably to the expert operator in the prediction of outcome of PULs. The model can be used by those with limited knowledge or understanding of the behaviour of serum biochemistry in the first trimester and in turn aids in the classification of PULs into those at low- and high risk for ectopic pregnancy (Figure 7.2).

Colleagues of varying clinical experience and levels of training can therefore use it in a multidisciplinary setting. This is especially the case in the ectopic pregnancy in the PUL population

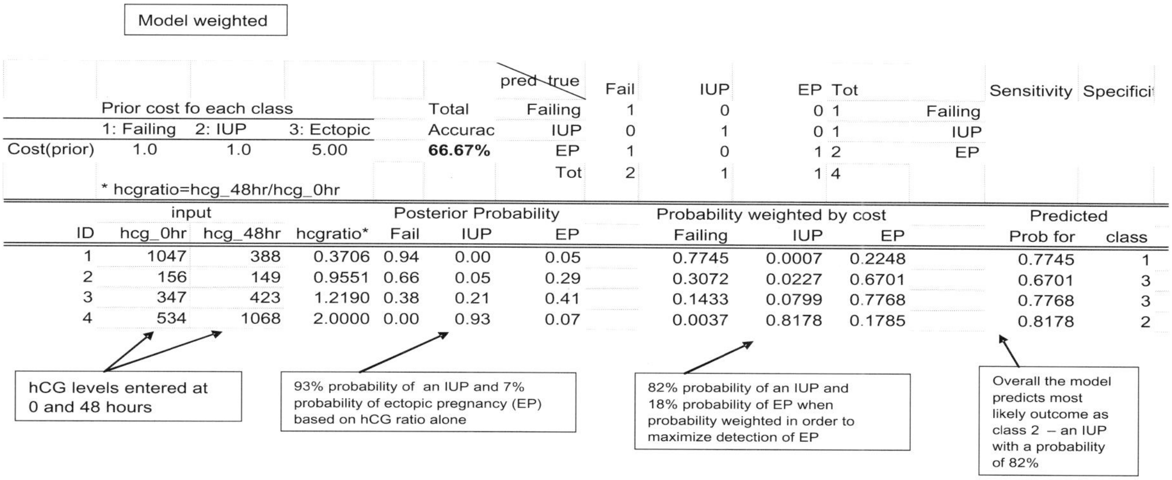

Model weighted						pred true	Fail	IUP	EP	Tot		Sensitivity	Specificit
	Prior cost fo each class				Total	Failing	1	0	0	1	Failing		
	1: Failing	2: IUP	3: Ectopic		Accurac	IUP	0	1	0	1	IUP		
Cost(prior)	1.0	1.0	5.00		**66.67%**	EP	1	0	1	2	EP		
						Tot	2	1	1	4			
	* hcgratio=hcg_48hr/hcg_0hr												

	input			Posterior Probability			Probability weighted by cost			Predicted	
ID	hcg_0hr	hcg_48hr	hcgratio*	Fail	IUP	EP	Failing	IUP	EP	Prob for	class
1	1047	388	0.3706	0.94	0.00	0.05	0.7745	0.0007	0.2248	0.7745	1
2	156	149	0.9551	0.66	0.05	0.29	0.3072	0.0227	0.6701	0.6701	3
3	347	423	1.2190	0.38	0.21	0.41	0.1433	0.0799	0.7768	0.7768	3
4	534	1068	2.0000	0.00	0.93	0.07	0.0037	0.8178	0.1785	0.8178	2

hCG levels entered at 0 and 48 hours

93% probability of an IUP and 7% probability of ectopic pregnancy (EP) based on hCG ratio alone

82% probability of an IUP and 18% probability of EP when probability weighted in order to maximize detection of EP

Overall the model predicts most likely outcome as class 2 – an IUP with a probability of 82%

Figure 7.2 Example of a mathematical model as it appeared on computer databases in the clinical setting. (Reproduced from Kirk et al., Ultrasound Obstet Gynecol 2006; 27:311–5, with permission John Wiley and Sons Ltd.)

whose heterogeneous biochemical behaviour can often result in misclassification, i.e. some ectopic pregnancies mimic failing PULs whilst others mimic ongoing intrauterine pregnancies. At present the number of follow up visits for women with a PUL is often protracted, especially in those women whose biochemistry does not conform to either a failing PUL or an intrauterine pregnancy. As this model classifies PULs at 48 hours there is also the potential to address this.

NEW MARKERS IN THE MANAGEMENT OF PREGNANCIES OF UNKNOWN LOCATION

In a further study, the use of maternal serum cancer antigen 125 (CA 125) and creatine kinase (CK) were evaluated in a PUL population.[20] The baseline serum levels of these biochemical markers did not differ significantly between the three outcome groups, i.e. the failing PULs, IUPs and ectopic pregnancies. This study concluded that absolute levels of serum CK and CA 125 at the defined times could not be used to predict the outcome of PULs.

UTERINE CURETTAGE IN THE MANAGEMENT OF PREGNANCIES OF UNKNOWN LOCATION

According to a Lancet review[21] on ectopic pregnancy, dilatation and curettage (D&C) can be safely performed only after a non-viable pregnancy has been documented by either a serum progesterone level of ≤15.9 nmol/L or the absence of a rise in serum hCG after 2 days; that is, an hCG ratio of <1.50. D&C would certainly be safe if the serum progesterone was <15.9 nmol/L, but in pregnancies that are already failing this seems unnecessary. Caution should be exercised in women whose hCG ratio is up to 1.50, as D&C in this situation may result in potential termination of early viable pregnancies.[22] Our unit certainly does not advocate the routine use of D&C in the management of women with a PUL.

CASE REPORT 1

A 32-year-old Para 0+1 woman with a previous history of ectopic pregnancy presented at 5+ weeks' gestation with light vaginal bleeding. She was clinically stable and TVS demonstrated a PUL. Serial hCG measurements at 0 and 48 h were 982 IU/L and 2000 IU/L, respectively. The hCG ratio was calculated to be 2.04 and she was classified as a low-risk PUL with follow-up scan arranged at 1 week. This scan demonstrated an early intrauterine gestational sac, thus confirming the location of the pregnancy. She was booked for a viability scan 2 weeks later.

CASE REPORT 2[23]

A 33-year-old Para 1 + 1 woman presented at 7 weeks' gestation with vaginal bleeding for 3 days. She had previously had one emergency Caesarean section at term. She was clinically stable and TVS demonstrated a PUL. Serial hCG measurements at 0 and 48 h were 112 IU/L and 113 IU/L, respectively. The hCG ratio was calculated to be 1.01 and the plan was to rescan her. She did not re-present until 10 days later, at which point her serum hCG was 126 IU/L. A repeat TVS was performed and she was noted to still have an empty uterus and the presence of a mass measuring 21 × 17 mm in the right ovary. A presumed diagnosis of an ovarian ectopic pregnancy was made and a repeat serum hCG level was scheduled for 48 h later. The hCG level (123 IU/L) had plateaued and as the woman was asymptomatic, intramuscular injection of methotrexate 50 mg/m^2 was given. Despite this treatment, the hCG levels continued to rise and 18 days later measured 214 IU/L. The scan was repeated and the right ovary was found to contain a highly vascularized 22 × 20 mm area, which at the time was thought to be 'highly suspicious' of an ovarian ectopic pregnancy. As the woman was still asymptomatic, it was decided to repeat the methotrexate. She was monitored closely as an outpatient, however her serum hCG level 12 days later was still rising (249 IU/L). A repeat TVS showed the right ovary to be grossly enlarged, 50 × 34 × 29 mm, and highly vascularized on colour Doppler. A germ cell tumour of the right ovary was considered and she was booked for laparoscopy and right salpingo-oophorectomy. Histology demonstrated a placental site trophoblastic tumour of the right ovary and fallopian tube. The woman was referred to the Trophoblastic Disease Screening and Treatment Centre at Charing Cross Hospital, London for follow up. Her serum hCG level was 2 IU/L 11 days post-surgery.

In our view, great care should be taken before giving medical treatment to a woman with a persisting PUL. When the location of the pregnancy cannot be identified by ultrasound and the serum hCG levels have reached a plateau, we recommend that a laparoscopy be performed prior to administering methotrexate therapy. When a woman denies any sexual relations in the presence of a positive pregnancy test, the possibility of hCG-secreting tumours must be entertained. This case highlights that a positive serum hCG does not always indicate pregnancy.

CONCLUSIONS

The prevalence of PULs is indirectly proportional to the quality of scanning for a given EPU. Most PULs are at low risk for an ectopic pregnancy provided that the ultrasound examiner is sufficiently skilled and uses an ultrasound system with acceptable image quality. Transvaginal ultrasound should be the primary non-invasive tool for the diagnosis of ectopic pregnancies. Uterine curettage should not be used in the routine management of PULs to distinguish an ectopic pregnancy from a miscarriage as there is potential to terminate ongoing viable pregnancies. Expectant management with biochemical follow up should be offered to women with a PUL if they are clinically stable. Based upon the interpretation of the hCG ratio (hCG 48 h/hCG 0 h) cut-offs, one can triage the PULs into low risk and high risk for ectopic pregnancy.

It is uncertain whether failing to diagnose the group of ectopic pregnancies in the PUL population is a problem, as not all ectopic pregnancies are dangerous and a proportion resolve spontaneously without intervention. To date, there is no way of predicting which ectopic pregnancies are likely to be self-limiting and which are likely to be dangerous. Even ectopic pregnancies with serum hCG levels lower than 10 IU/L can rupture. The unpredictable nature of ectopic pregnancies emphasizes the need for the development of mathematical models which not only have the potential to predict this subgroup of PULs (see Figure 7.1), but also decrease the number of follow up visits to make the diagnosis. The future management of women with PULs will centre on reducing follow-up visits without compromising safety.

PRACTICAL POINTS

1. Most PULs are at low risk for an ectopic pregnancy provided that the ultrasound examiner is sufficiently skilled and uses an ultrasound system with acceptable image quality.
2. Evaluation of serum hormone levels at defined times in women with a PUL can be used reliably to predict immediately viability of a PUL, but cannot predict its location.
3. Traditional hormonal criteria for the prediction of ectopic pregnancy in a PUL population perform poorly.
4. The accuracy of the discriminatory zone for the detection of ectopic pregnancies in specialist scanning units is much lower than in non-scanning-based units.
5. As the prevalence of ectopic pregnancies in a PUL population increases, so too does the effectiveness of the discriminatory zone.
6. An hCG ratio cut-off <0.87 or serum progesterone measurement alone can be used to identify spontaneously resolving pregnancies in a PUL population.
7. The logistic regression model M1, based on the hCG ratio, not only predicts the ectopic pregnancy group but also the failing PUL and the intrauterine pregnancy groups in a PUL population.
8. This model, M1, compares favourably to the expert operator in the prediction of outcome of PULs.
9. Absolute levels of serum CK and CA 125 at the defined times cannot be used to predict the outcome of PULs.
10. The performance of any mathematical model is dependent on the diagnostic accuracy of the final clinical outcomes, i.e. the failing PULs, intrauterine pregnancies, ectopic pregnancies and persisting PULs.
11. In most cases, uterine curettage should not play a role in the classification of PULs.
12. The future management of women with PULs will centre on reducing follow up visits without compromising safety.

REFERENCES

1. Condous G, Lu C, Van Huffel S, Timmerman D, Bourne T. Human chorionic gonadotrophin and progesterone levels for the investigation of pregnancies of unknown location. Int J Gynecol Obstet 2004; 86:351–7.
2. Cacciatore B, Stenman UH, Ylostalo P. Diagnosis of ectopic pregnancy by vaginal ultrasonography in combination with a discriminatory serum hCG level of 1000 IU/L (IRP). Br J Obstet Gynaecol 1990; 97:904–8.
3. Hahlin M, Thorburn J, Bryman I. The expectant management of early pregnancies of uncertain site. Hum Reprod 1995; 10:1223–7.
4. Banerjee S, Aslam N, Zosmer N, et al. The expectant management of women with pregnancies of unknown location. Ultrasound Obstet Gynecol 1999; 14:231–6.
5. Cacciatore B, Ylostalo P, Stenman UH, et al. Suspected ectopic pregnancy: ultrasound findings and hCG levels assessed by an immunofluorometric assay. Br J Obstet Gynaecol 1988; 95:497–502.
6. Banerjee S, Aslam N, Woelfer B, et al. Expectant management of early pregnancies of unknown location: a prospective evaluation of methods to predict spontaneous resolution of pregnancy. Br J Obstet Gynaecol 2001; 108:158–63.
7. Hajenius PJ, Mol BW, Ankum WM, et al. Suspected ectopic pregnancy: expectant management in patients with negative sonographic findings and low serum hCG concentrations. Early Pregnancy 1995; 1:258–62.
8. Mol BW, Hajenius PJ, Engelsbel S, et al. Serum human chorionic gonadotropin measurement in the diagnosis of ectopic pregnancy when transvaginal sonography is inconclusive. Fertil Steril 1998; 70:972–81.
9. Ankum WM, Van der Veen F, Hamerlynck JVThH, et al. Transvaginal sonography and human chorionic gonadotrophin measurements in suspected ectopic pregnancy: a detailed analysis of a diagnostic approach. Hum Reprod 993; 8:1307–11.
10. Condous G, Kirk E, Lu C, et al. What is the diagnostic accuracy of varying discriminatory zones for the prediction of ectopic pregnancy in women with a pregnancy of unknown location. Ultrasound Obstet Gynecol 2005; 26:770–5.
11. Condous G, Okaro E, Khalid A, et al. The use of a new logistic regression model for predicting the outcome of pregnancies of unknown location. Hum Reprod 2004; 19:1900–10.

12. Condous G, Kirk E, Van Calster B, et al. Failing pregnancies of unknown location: a prospective evaluation of the human chorionic gonadotrophin ratio. Br J Obstets Gynaecol, 2006; 113:521–7.

13. Ling FW, Stovall TG. Update on the diagnosis and management of ectopic pregnancy. In: Advances in Obstetrics and Gynecology, 1. Chicago: Mosby Year Book, 1994: 55–83.

14. Kadar N, Caldwell BV, Romero R. A method of screening for ectopic pregnancy and its indications. Obstet Gynecol 1981; 58:162–6.

15. Barnhart KT, Simhan H, Kamelle SA. Diagnostic accuracy of ultrasound above and below the beta-hCG discriminatory zone. Obstet Gynecol 1999; 94:583–7.

16. Mol B, Van der Veen F. Role of transvaginal ultrasonography in the diagnosis of ectopic pregnancy. Fertil Steril 1998; 70:594–5.

17. Ankum W, Hajenius P, Schrevel L, et al. Management of suspected ectopic pregnancy: impact of new diagnostic tools in 686 consecutive cases. J Reprod Med 1996; 41:724–8.

18. Mol BW, Hajenius PJ, Engelsbel S, et al. Are gestational age and endometrial thickness alternatives for serum human chorionic gonadotropin as criteria for the diagnosis of ectopic pregnancy? Fertil Steril 1999; 72:643–5.

19. Kirk E, Condous G, Haider Z, et al. The practical application of a mathematical model to predict the outcome of pregnancies of unknown location (PULs). Ultrasound Obstet Gynecol 2006; in press.

20. Condous G, Kirk E, Syed A, et al. Do levels of serum cancer antigen 125 and creatine kinase predict the outcome in pregnancies of unknown location? Hum Reprod 2005; 20:3348–54.

21. Pisarska M, Carson S, Buster J. Ectopic pregnancy. Lancet 1998; 351:1115–20.

22. Condous G, Kirk E, Lu C et al. There is no role for uterine curettage in women with a pregnancy of unknown location. Hum Reprod 2006; in press.

23. Condous G, Thomas J, Okaro E, Bourne T. Placental site trophoblastic tumor masquerading as an ovarian ectopic pregnancy. Ultrasound Obstet Gynecol 2003; 21:504–6.

8

The use of ultrasound to diagnose tubal ectopic pregnancy

George Condous

Introduction • Laparoscopy versus transvaginal ultrasound • Other ultrasonographic markers • Heterotopic pregnancy • Should we screen women for ectopic pregnancy? • Timing of the first ultrasound scan • Case report 1 • Case report 2 • Conclusions • Practical points

INTRODUCTION

It used to be standard teaching that an 'empty uterus with a positive pregnancy test is an ectopic pregnancy until proved otherwise'. This was based on transabdominal ultrasound findings and usually led to the patient being admitted for laparoscopy. We have seen in Chapter 2 that an intrauterine pregnancy can be visualized at a very early stage. However today if a pregnancy cannot be seen on transvaginal ultrasonography the situation is described as a pregnancy of unknown location (PUL) and the management is described in detail in Chapter 7. The diagnosis of a tubal ectopic pregnancy should instead be based upon the positive visualization of an adnexal mass using transvaginal ultrasonography (TVS). This does not require particularly sophisticated equipment and conventional two-dimensional grey-scale imaging alone is sufficient to make the diagnosis. Neither three-dimensional ultrasound nor colour Doppler is required. Although TVS has its obvious benefits, surgery should not be delayed in women who are haemodynamically unstable in order to confirm the diagnosis using ultrasound. Common sense must be applied and some patients will need to go straight to the operating theatre on the basis of the clinical findings alone.

All women with a positive pregnancy test and lower abdominal pain with or without vaginal bleeding should undergo an ultrasound scan in order to locate the pregnancy. In most cases, if an ectopic pregnancy is present it will be visible on ultrasound. In a recent study in our unit, 90.9% of ectopic pregnancies were correctly identified prior to surgery using TVS alone.[1] This high sensitivity has been previously demonstrated with between 87% and 93% of ectopic pregnancies being identified using TVS prior to surgery.[2,3] With proper training in ultrasonography and quality control these high standards are achievable.

In the absence of an intrauterine sac, the adnexae must be carefully examined in order to exclude or diagnose an ectopic pregnancy. The diagnosis of an ectopic pregnancy is made if one of the following grey-scale appearances are present: (1) an inhomogeneous mass or blob sign adjacent to and moving separately to the ovary[1] (Figure 8.1); or (2) a mass with a hyperechoic ring around the gestational sac or bagel sign[1] (Figure 8.2); or (3) a gestational sac with a fetal pole with cardiac activity, i.e. a viable extrauterine pregnancy[1] (Figure 8.3); or (4) a

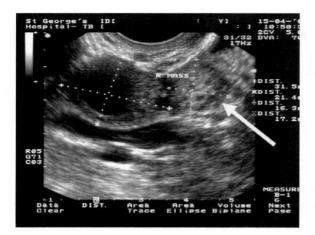

Figure 8.1 Tubal ectopic pregnancy; the solid arrow depicts an inhomogeneous mass or 'blob sign' on transvaginal scan. (Reproduced with permission from Condous et al. Ultrasound Obstet Gynecol 2003; 2:420–30.)

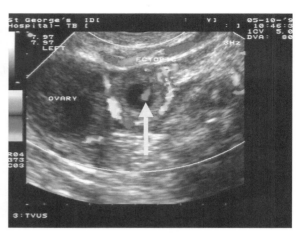

Figure 8.3 Viable tubal ectopic pregnancy; solid arrow points to fetal cardiac activity demonstrated with colour Doppler. (See also colour plate)

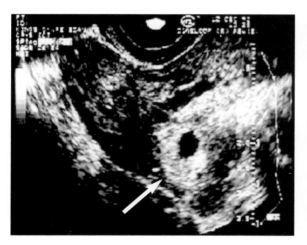

Figure 8.2 Transvaginal scan image demonstrating 'bagel' sign. The solid arrow shows ectopic pregnancy characterized by the 'bagel sign'. (Reproduced with permission from Condous et al. Ultrasound Obstet Gynecol 2003; 2:420–30.)

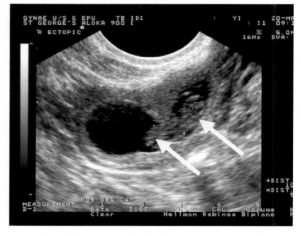

Figure 8.4 Twin non-viable tubal ectopic pregnancy. Solid arrows point to both fetal poles.

gestational sac with a fetal pole without cardiac activity, i.e. a non-viable extrauterine pregnancy[1] (Figure 8.4). A recent study confirmed previously published data relating to the characteristic appearances of ectopic pregnancy on TVS. The majority of confirmed ectopic pregnancies were seen as an inhomogeneous mass or 'blob' (57.9%). A total of 20.4% were visualized as a hyperechoic ring and only 13.2% were visualized as a gestational sac with a fetal pole and 55% of these had positive fetal cardiac activity.[1] Misdiagnosis using TVS should be relatively uncommon and in this study the false positive rate was only 5.9%.

Using meta-analysis, Brown and Doubilet evaluated the performance of TVS for the diagnosis of ectopic pregnancy.[4] Ten studies involving 2216 women, 565 with ectopic pregnancy, were included in the analysis. Four different ultrasonographic criteria were assessed as follows: criterion A, a gestational sac with a fetal pole with cardiac activity, i.e. a viable extrauterine pregnancy; criterion B, a gestational sac with a fetal pole without cardiac activity, i.e. a non-viable extrauterine pregnancy; criterion C, a mass with a hyperechoic ring around the gestational sac, i.e. an empty 'tubal ring'; and criterion D, an inhomogeneous adnexal mass or blob sign. The positive predictive values (PPV) for criteria A, B and C were 97.8 to 100%. In the study by Condous et al., the PPV for criteria A, B and C were 100%, in keeping with these data, whilst the PPV for criterion D was 88.6% compared with 96.3% in Brown and Doubilet's study.[1] This high predictive value of TVS for the diagnosis of ectopic pregnancy has made a significant difference to patient management. As will be described in later chapters, the positive finding of an ectopic pregnancy using ultrasound does not require laparoscopic confirmation and expectant or medical management can be initiated without further intervention.

LAPAROSCOPY VERSUS TRANSVAGINAL ULTRASOUND

Laparoscopy has always been considered the gold standard for the diagnosis of ectopic pregnancy.[5] Laparoscopy, however, does not confer 100% sensitivity, and false-negative laparoscopies do occur. These may occur when early ongoing ectopic pregnancies are too small to be seen or when some ectopic pregnancies resolve spontaneously and are never seen. There are even rarer instances where a fallopian tube is removed at the time of laparoscopy for possible ectopic pregnancy, only to show no chorionic villi on subsequent histology. TVS and serum human chorionic gonadotrophin (hCG) measurements have been shown to be very reliable for the diagnosis of ectopic pregnancies.[6] Given the current trends towards conservative management described in

Chapters 9 and 10, it is perhaps time to recognize that transvaginal ultrasound can also be used as a standard on which to judge the presence or absence of an ectopic pregnancy. Despite this, in many units the diagnosis of ectopic pregnancy is not usually made based on ultrasound signs alone, despite the data described above that demonstrate the capability of TVS as a single test to positively identify an ectopic pregnancy.[1] The presence or absence of an ectopic pregnancy seen on scan alongside levels of serum hCG should be used as a basis on which treatment decisions are made. Laparoscopy should not be considered a diagnostic tool in the majority of cases, but seen as something that facilitates surgical treatment.

OTHER ULTRASONOGRAPHIC MARKERS

These markers for ectopic pregnancies include the corpus luteum and/or the presence of blood in the pelvis. The corpus luteum can be a potential guide to the location of the ectopic pregnancy as it will be on the ipsilateral side in 70–85% of cases.[1,7,8] Ectopic pregnancy associated with haemoperitoneum on TVS suggests the possibility of tubal rupture, and this situation requires surgical intervention in the majority of cases; however, although the incidence of haemoperitoneum is between 18% and 34%,[1,9,10] this does not invariably mean that tubal rupture has occurred. Most ectopic pregnancies with blood in the pouch of Douglas have 'leakage' from the lumen of the fimbrial end of the fallopian tube. It is very difficult to quantify the volume of haemoperitoneum on ultrasound scan, however the presence of blood in Morrison's pouch can be used as a marker for more significant haemoperitoneum. Morrison's pouch is easily demonstrated on a transabdominal scan if there is significant fluid in the abdomen and pelvis and in the space between Gerota's fascia surrounding the kidney and Glisson's capsule of the liver.

HETEROTOPIC PREGNANCY

Spontaneous heterotopic pregnancy is rare and is reported to occur in between 1:10 000 and 1:50 000 pregnancies (Figure 8.5).[11] They are

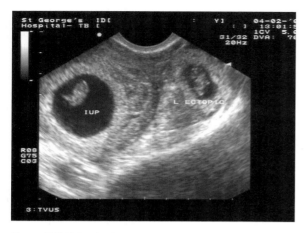

Figure 8.5 Heterotopic pregnancy – spontaneous conception. (Reproduced with permission from Condous et al. Best Pract Res Clin Obstet Gynaecol, 2004; 18:37–57.)

often missed as once an intrauterine pregnancy has been visualized it is often assumed that an ectopic pregnancy cannot be present. However women who have undergone assisted reproductive techniques (ARTs) have an incidence of heterotopic pregnancy as high as 1%.[11] Therefore, if an intrauterine sac is confirmed on TVS in these women, the adnexae must be carefully inspected to exclude tubal pathology. In women who have undergone ARTs, even with a confirmed intrauterine gestational sac, if they have ongoing abdominal pain with or without haemodynamic compromise, a heterotopic pregnancy should always be considered. These pregnancies do represent a management problem. Conservative management is difficult as hCG levels cannot be interpreted in the presence of a viable intrauterine pregnancy and surgery is usually the treatment of choice.

SHOULD WE SCREEN WOMEN FOR ECTOPIC PREGNANCY?

Screening for ectopic pregnancies in asymptomatic women at earlier gestations is not generally advised in the low risk population. Although scanning and diagnosing all women with ectopic pregnancies at much earlier gesta-

tions would be the ideal scenario, such a policy would result in more women having an inconclusive scan known as a pregnancy of unknown location. This in turn would result in an increased number of subsequent scans and follow-up visits for the women. This would have financial implications on any EPU, not to mention the possible psychological morbidity for the women. In contrast those women who have had a previous ectopic pregnancy or a significant risk factor for the disease should be asked to attend for an early scan.

TIMING OF THE FIRST ULTRASOUND SCAN

The timing of the first trimester scan is important. If carried out too early is will lead to inconclusive results and increased anxiety. Some units in the United Kingdom do not offer ultrasound scans to women in the first trimester until after 7 weeks' gestation. Such a policy sets a dangerous precedent as one cannot rely on the last menstrual period to determine whether a woman should undergo a scan or not, not to mention the fact that many ectopic pregnancies present before this gestation. In a recent study, women with lower abdominal pain and a history of ectopic pregnancy presented at a mean gestation of 20 days![1]

CASE REPORT 1

A 26-year-old Para 0+0 woman presented with right iliac fossa pain and a positive urinary pregnancy test at 7 weeks' gestation according to her last menstrual period. A TVS at the time demonstrated a right adnexal 'blob' sign measuring 23 × 27 mm with an ipsilateral corpus luteum. She was also noted to have free fluid in the pouch of Douglas that was ground glass in appearance. Her serum hCG level was 2345 IU/L and a diagnosis of a right sided tubal ectopic pregnancy with haemoperitoneum was made. In view of her symptomatology and scan findings she was managed surgically and underwent a laparoscopic linear salpingotomy. She was followed up with weekly serum hCG levels to exclude persistent trophoblastic disease and was discharged when her serum hCG was <10 IU/L after 3 weeks.

CASE REPORT 2

A 34-year-old Para 2+0 woman presented at 8 weeks' gestation with central lower abdominal pain and heavy vaginal bleeding with clots. TVS demonstrated an empty uterus with an endometrial thickness of 10 mm, no adnexal mass of note and no haemoperitoneum. Although a diagnosis of a 'complete miscarriage'' was made on the basis of history and scan findings, she was followed up with serial biochemistry at 0 h and 48 h. Her serum hCG and progesterone levels at presentation were 847 IU/L and 34 nmol/L, respectively. Subsequent serum hCG level at 48 h was not falling and had increased to 1226 IU/L. She was therefore recalled for a scan and at the time found to be stable and relatively asymptomatic. TVS demonstrated a left-sided adnexal mass with bagel sign measuring 22 × 19 mm – there was no haemoperitoneum. She was counselled about the treatment options and thereafter managed successfully with methotrexate. All women with a 'complete miscarriage' should be managed in the same way as a PUL, i.e. with serial hCG follow up to confirm the diagnosis. If hCG levels rise instead of fall, then ultrasound scan is essential to establish the diagnosis.

CONCLUSIONS

Ultrasound, and in particular TVS, has resulted in more ectopic pregnancies being diagnosed at earlier gestations in clinically stable women. Consequently more conservative treatment options are available to both the gynaecologist and the woman. TVS has revolutionized the non-invasive diagnosis of ectopic pregnancy. Ectopic pregnancy diagnosis should be based on the positive visualization of an adnexal mass using TVS. Of women who present with an ectopic pregnancy 90.9% can be diagnosed directly using ultrasound as a single stand-alone test.

PRACTICAL POINTS

1. Transvaginal and not transabdominal ultrasonography should be used when diagnosing ectopic pregnancy.
2. The vast majority of ectopic pregnancies can be visualized prior to surgery using TVS alone.
3. The most common sonographic appearance of an ectopic pregnancy on 2-D ultrasound is a small inhomogeneous mass or 'blob sign'.
4. All women, regardless of LMP, who present in the first trimester with lower abdominal pain with or without vaginal bleeding must be scanned.
5. In women who have undergone ARTs, with a confirmed intrauterine gestational sac on TVS, and ongoing abdominal pain with or without haemodynamic compromise, always consider a heterotopic pregnancy.
6. The diagnosis of a complete miscarriage on the basis of history and scan findings alone is unreliable. A small but significant proportion of these women will have an underlying ectopic pregnancy and therefore serial hCG follow up is essential.

REFERENCES

1. Condous G, Okaro E, Khalid A, et al. The accuracy of transvaginal ultrasonography for the diagnosis of ectopic pregnancy prior to surgery. Hum Reprod 2005; 20:1404–9.
2. Cacciatore B, Stenman UH, Ylostalo P. Diagnosis of ectopic pregnancy by vaginal ultrasonography in combination with a discriminatory serum hCG level of 1000 IU/L (IRP). Br J Obstet Gynaecol 1990; 97:904–8.
3. Shalev E, Yarom I, Bustan M, et al. Transvaginal sonography as the ultimate diagnostic tool for the management of ectopic pregnancy: experience with 840 cases. Fertil Steril 1998; 69:62–5.
4. Brown DL, Doubilet PM. Transvaginal sonography for diagnosing ectopic pregnancy: positivity criteria and

performance characteristics. J Ultrasound Med 1994; 13:259–66.

5. Ankum WM, Van der Veen F, Hamerlynck JV, et al. Laparoscopy: a dispensable tool in the diagnosis of ectopic pregnancy? Hum Reprod 1993; 8:1301–6.

6. Ankum WM, Van der Veen F, Hamerlynck JV, et al. Transvaginal sonography and human chorionic gonadotrophin measurements in suspected ectopic pregnancy: a detailed analysis of a diagnostic approach. Hum Reprod 1993; 8:1307–11.

7. Walters MD, Eddy C, Pauerstein CJ. The contralateral corpus luteum and tubal pregnancy. Obstet Gynecol 1987; 70:823–6.

8. Jurkovic D, Bourne TH, Jauniaux E, et al. Transvaginal color Doppler study of blood flow in ectopic pregnancies. Fertil Steril 1992; 57:68–73.

9. DiMarchi JM, Kosasa TS, Hale RW. What is the significance of the human chorionic gonadotropin value in ectopic pregnancy? Obstets Gynecol 1989; 74:851–5.

10. Saxon D, Falcone T, Mascha EJ, et al. A study of ruptured tubal ectopic pregnancy. Obstets Gynecol 1997; 90:6–9.

11. Condous G, Okaro E, Bourne T. The conservative management of early pregnancy complications: a review of the literature. Ultrasound Obstet Gynecol 2003; 22:420–30.

9

The expectant management of ectopic pregnancy

Emma Kirk

Introduction • Success rates • Predictors of success • Reproductive outcome • Comparison to medical management • Suggested management protocol • Case report 1 • Case report 2 • Practical points

INTRODUCTION

Not all ectopic pregnancies need intervention – either in the form of surgery or medical management. As we have already seen in Chapter 8, advances in high-quality ultrasound mean that many ectopic pregnancies can be detected at an early stage; however, many of these will be pregnancies that are destined to fail. In the past, many of these ectopic pregnancies would have gone undetected. However they create a management problem in that these women may be subjected to unnecessary surgery or medical therapy for a self-limiting condition.

Expectant management can be an appropriate and successful management option for those ectopic pregnancies which are destined to fail. The difficulty is in predicting which ectopic pregnancies are likely to undergo successful spontaneous resolution. This chapter aims to give an overview of the use of expectant management in the treatment of tubal ectopic pregnancies.

SUCCESS RATES

Reported success rates for expectant management vary from 48 to 100%.[1–8] Table 9.1 summarizes studies published between 1992 and 2004.[9]

The largest study to date is on 118 ectopic pregnancies. In this particular study, the overall success rate for expectant management was 65.3% (77/118).[2] Transvaginal ultrasound scans (TVS) and serum hCG determinations were performed every 1–3 days until the hCG was less than 10 IU/L. The mean time to resolution was 20 days (range 4–67 days). The initial serum hCG level was much lower in those with successful expectant management compared to those with failed expectant management, 374 IU/L (range, 20–10 762 IU/L) compared to 741 IU/L (range, 165–14 047 IU/L). An estimate of the likely success of an expectant management strategy can be made on the basis of a single measurement of serum hCG. There was an 88% success rate when the initial hCG level was <200 IU/L but only 25% at levels of >2000 IU/L. A more recently published study has shown similar success rates, with 96% success when the hCG was <175 IU/L.[8] However, limiting expectant management to ectopic pregnancies with such relatively low hCG levels would restrict this approach to only a few cases.

Different inclusion criteria for expectant management led to variations in success rates. For example some studies include pregnancies of unknown location (PULs) rather than laparoscopically or sonographically visualized ectopic

Table 9.1. Expectant management: inclusion criteria and short-term outcome

Author and reference	Year	n =	Overall success	Mean hCG – success (IU/L)	Mean hCG – failure (IU/L)	Time to resolution (days)	Comments on entry criteria	Other comments
Ylostalo[1]	1992	83	69% (57/83)				• Decreasing hCG	
Korhonen[2]	1994	118	65.3% (77/118)	374 (20–10 762)	741 (165–14 047)	20 (4–67)		• 88% success if hCG <200 IU/L • 25% success if hCG >2000 IU/L
Cacciatore[3]	1995	71	69% (49/71)	583 (64–2542)	470 (161–2525)	25 (8–60)	• Decrease in hCG over 48 hours • Adnexal mass <5 cm diameter	
Trio[3]	1995	67	73% (49/67)	455 (36–16 400)	2000 (93–22 300)	31 ± 19	• 39% not positively identified on TVS • Ectopic <4 cm diameter	• 88% success if hCG <1000 IU/L
Shalev[5]	1995	60	47.7% (28/60)				• Confirmed laparoscopically • Declining hCG level	• 60% success if hCG <2000 IU/L • 7% success if hCG >2000 IU/L
Lui[6]	1997	17	100% (17/17)			17	• Tubal diameter <3 cm • Free fluid <100 ml • No fetal cardiac activity • Haemodynamic stability	
Olofsson[7]	2001	17	82.4% (14/17)					
Elson[8]	2004	107	70% (75/107)	246 (99–536)	628 (254–1402)	15 (3–66)	• Haemodynamic stability • No fetal cardiac activity • No haemoperitoneum	• 96% success if hCG <175 IU/L • 66% success if hCG 175–1500 IU/L • 21% success if hCG >1500 IU/L • 0% success if hCG >1500 IU/L and >42 days pregnant

From Kirk E, Condous G, Bourne T. Non-surgical management of ectopic pregnancy.[9]

pregnancies. There is no doubt that this group will contain some ectopic pregnancies but it may also contain some missed failed intrauterine pregnancies. The number of ectopic pregnancies in a population of PULs has been reported to be as low as 7–8%.[10,11] In the majority of studies, a single cut-off level of serum hCG has been used as the main criterion for inclusion. Selection for expectant management on the basis of single serum hCG and progesterone levels will lead to variations in success rates. Units only managing ectopic pregnancies expectantly with very low hCG levels (e.g. <200 IU/L) are likely to have much higher success rates than if a higher cut-off hCG level is used. Exclusion criteria that have been cited for expectant management include an ectopic mass of >3 cm, haemoperitoneum, positive fetal cardiac activity, pain and an increasing hCG level. Not all of these are absolute contraindications and each case must be judged on its merits.

PREDICTORS OF SUCCESS

Investigators have looked at gestation, ultrasound findings and serum biochemistry to try to establish likely predictors of success for expectant management. The following have been found to be significant predictors of success: lower initial hCG levels, a decreasing trend in hCG levels over time, the absence of a visible ectopic gestation sac and a longer time from the last menstrual period.[4,12] Serum hCG cut-off levels vary, but in one study an initial hCG level of <1000 IU/L was chosen as the optimal cut off and was found to identify 88% of women destined to have spontaneous resolution of the ectopic pregnancy.[4] The success rate was only 48% when the serum hCG was >1000 IU/L.

Serial TVS monitoring of ectopic pregnancies selected for expectant management, appears useful in recognizing which ones are most likely to resolve spontaneously. One study has shown that 55% of ectopic pregnancies managed successfully had decreased in size by 3 days and 84% by 7 days.[3] A decrease in ectopic size at day 7 had a sensitivity of 84% and a specificity of 100% for the prediction of spontaneous resolution.

REPRODUCTIVE OUTCOME

Subsequent fertility is an important long-term outcome. Hysterosalpingography performed after expectant management has shown patency in the affected tube in up to 93% of cases.[13] Intrauterine pregnancy rates of 63–88% have been seen following expectant management of ectopic pregnancy.[13–16] A subsequent ectopic pregnancy has been seen in 4–5% of cases.[13,14]

A study has shown similar intrauterine pregnancy rates in those managed expectantly with ectopic pregnancy (63%) compared to those managed surgically (51%).[15] Interestingly, those undergoing delayed surgery due to failure of initial expectant management had similar subsequent intrauterine conception rates to those that underwent primary surgery.[15]

COMPARISON TO MEDICAL MANAGEMENT

Expectant management has been compared to systemic methotrexate. Sixty haemodynamically stable women were randomized to 5 days of treatment with either 2.5 mg/day of oral methotrexate or placebo.[17] The overall success rate was 77% with no significant differences in primary treatment success between the two methods. At present there are no other published randomized controlled studies comparing either expectant management to systemic medical treatment or surgery.

SUGGESTED MANAGEMENT PROTOCOL

As for medical management of ectopic pregnancies, units offering expectant management should have clear protocols including details of inclusion and exclusion criteria and the follow up needed. It is also essential that women undergoing such management have access 24 hours a day to healthcare professionals if any problems arise. Expectant management may involve multiple clinic visits to monitor serum hCG levels. Ectopic pregnancies can rupture despite decreasing and low hCG levels, so hCG levels must be monitored until they are less than 15 IU/L. If there are any doubts about a woman's compliance with follow up, the decision to manage her ectopic pregnancy expectantly should be re-evaluated.

After the ultrasound diagnosis of an ectopic pregnancy, a bimanual examination should be performed. If there is no cervical excitation or adnexal tenderness, and the woman is pain-free and haemodynamically stable with no evidence of fetal cardiac activity or haemoperitoneum on TVS, expectant management can be considered. Blood should be taken for serum hCG and progesterone, a full blood count and group and save. Units will use different cut-off levels of initial hCG, for example 3000 IU/L or 5000 IU/L for expectant management. In general women with an initial hCG of 1000 IU/L that decreases over 48 hours are good candidates for expectant management. We believe that there is an argument for repeating the hCG level at 48 hours before deciding on a management plan, in order to calculate the pretreatment hCG ratio (hCG 48 h/hCG 0 h). If the hCG ratio is less than 0.8, there is an 80% chance of successful expectant management.[18] The majority of women managed expectantly should be able to remain as outpatients. Serum hCG levels should be checked every 48 hours for the first week or at least until there is more than a 20% decrease in 48 hours. Levels should then be checked weekly until less than 15 IU/L. If the levels do not decrease, the woman should be reviewed as to whether methotrexate treatment is indicated or surgery should be performed. In the course of follow up, if the woman develops any pain she should be reviewed immediately with a repeat transvaginal ultrasound examination, bimanual examination, serum hCG and full blood count. The findings of a small amount of haemoperitoneum in a haemodynamically stable woman with minimal pain and a stable haemoglobin level, could indicate possible tubal miscarriage. In these cases further expectant management as an inpatient with monitoring of hCG levels may be possible. If there is any severe pain, haemodynamic instability or a large amount of haemoperitoneum on TVS, tubal rupture cannot be excluded and so a laparoscopy should be performed and then a salpingectomy or salpingotomy performed if necessary.

Figure 10.1 (p. 91) shows a suggested conservative management protocol for ectopic pregnancy.

CASE REPORT 1

A 31-year-old woman presented to the EPU in her first pregnancy with some light vaginal bleeding. She was 13 weeks' gestation according to her last menstrual period. It was an unplanned pregnancy. She had previously had some light vaginal bleeding and had had an abdominal scan at a termination clinic 2 weeks previously which had showed possible retained products of conception. A TVS was performed which showed a 19 × 16 × 15 mm left adnexal inhomogeneous mass. There was no free fluid, and no pain or tenderness elicited on TVS. She was given the diagnosis of a left tubal ectopic pregnancy. Blood was taken. The initial serum hCG was 1286 IU/L and the progesterone 6 nmol/L. As she was haemodynamically stable and asymptomatic, the decision was made to repeat the hCG level in 48 hours. The hCG was 962 IU/L at 48 hours (hCG ratio 0.75) and the progesterone 5 nmol/L. The hCG was checked every 48 hours until day 7 and then weekly. The ectopic pregnancy was successfully managed expectantly, with the hCG level <15 IU/L within 66 days of initial presentation to the EPU (Figure 9.1).

CASE REPORT 2

A 27-year-old woman attended the EPU with a 2-week history of cramp-like lower abdominal pain and light vaginal spotting. It was her first pregnancy and she was 8 weeks and 2 days' gestation according to her last menstrual period. A TVS was performed which showed an empty uterus with a small right-sided inhomogeneous mass measuring 15 × 16 × 15 mm, next to the right ovary. There was a small amount of anechoic free fluid in the pouch of Douglas. There was no pelvic tenderness on vaginal examination. Bloods were taken. The serum hCG was 320 IU/L and the progesterone was 7 nmol/L. The decision was made to repeat the bloods in 48 hours. At 48 hours the hCG had decreased to 240 IU/L (hCG

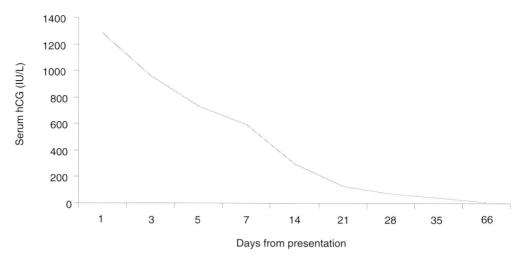

Figure 9.1 Graph showing a spontaneous decrease in hCG levels in an expectantly managed ectopic pregnancy

ratio 0.75), so the decision was made to manage expectantly. The bloods were repeated at 96 hours. The hCG at 96 hours was now 295 IU/L and the progesterone level was 5 nmol/L. As the levels had increased the decision was made to give a single dose of systemic methotrexate (50 mg/m²). Serum hCG follow up was performed using the single-dose methotrexate protocol. The hCG decreased only 10% between days 4 and 7, so a second dose was administered. Following the second dose the hCG decreased to <15 IU/L within 3 weeks of follow up. A repeat scan 3 months post treatment showed no obvious residual ectopic mass.

PRACTICAL POINTS

1. Expectant management is safe and effective for a select group of women.
2. Decreasing and low hCG levels (<1000 IU/L) are associated with successful outcome.
3. An hCG ratio of less than 0.8 is associated with a high success rate for expectant management.
4. Close follow up is essential.

REFERENCES

1. Ylostalo P, Cacciatore B, Sjoberg J, et al. Expectant management of ectopic pregnancy. Obstet Gynecol 1992; 80:345–8.
2. Korhonen J, Stenman UH, Ylostalo P. Serum human chorionic gonadotrophin dynamics during spontaneous resolution of ectopic pregnancy. Fertil Steril 1994; 61:632–6.
3. Cacciatore B, Korhonen J, Stenman UH, Ylostalo P. Transvaginal sonography and serum hCG in monitoring of presumed ectopic pregnancies selected for expectant management. Ultrasound Obstet Gynecol 1995; 5:297–300.
4. Trio D, Strobelt N, Picciolo C, Lapinski RH, Ghidini A. Prognostic factors for successful expectant management of ectopic pregnancy. Fertil Steril 1995; 63: 469–72.
5. Shalev E, Peleg D, Tsabari A, Romano S, Bustan M. Spontaneous resolution of ectopic tubal pregnancy: natural history. Fertil Steril 1995; 63:15–9.
6. Lui A, D'Ottavio G, Rustico MA, et al . Conservative management of ectopic pregnancy. Minerva Ginecol 1997; 49:67–72.

7. Olofsson JI, Poromaa IS, Ottander U, et al. Clinical and pregnancy outcome following ectopic pregnancy; a prospective study comparing expectancy, surgery and systemic methotrexate treatment. Acta Obstet Gynecol Scand 2001; 80:744–9.

8. Elson J, Tailor A, Banerjee S, et al. Expectant management of tubal ectopic pregnancy: prediction of successful outcome using decision tree analysis. Ultrasound Obstet Gynecol 2004; 23:552–6.

9. Kirk E, Condous G, Bourne T. The non-surgical management of ectopic pregnancy. Ultrasound Obstet Gynecol 2006; 27:91–100.

10. Condous G, Okaro E, Khalid A, et al. The use of a new logistic regression model for predicting the outcome of pregnancies of unknown location. Hum Reprod 2004; 19:1900–10.

11. Banerjee S, Aslam N, Woefler B, et al. Expectant management of early pregnancies of unknown location: a prospective evaluation of methods to predict spontaneous resolution of pregnancy. Br J Obstet Gynaecol 2001; 108:158–3.

12. Atri M, Chow CM, Kintzen G, et al. Expectant treatment of ectopic pregnancies: clinical and sonographic predictors. Am J Roentgenol 2001; 176:123–7.

13. Rantala M, Makinen J. Tubal patency and fertility outcome after expectant management of ectopic pregnancy. Fertil Steril 1997; 68:1043–6.

14. Zohav E, Gemer O, Segal S. Reproductive outcome after expectant management of ectopic pregnancy. Eur J Obstet Gynecol Reprod Biol 1996; 66:1–2.

15. Strobelt N, Mariani E, Ferrari L, et al. Fertility after ectopic pregnancy. Effects of surgery and expectant management. J Reprod Med 2000; 45(10):803–7.

16. Fernandez H, Lelaidier C, Baton C, et al. Return of reproductive performance after expectant management and local treatment for ectopic pregnancy. Hum Reprod 1991; 6:1474–7.

17. Korhonen J, Stenman UH, Ylostalo P. Low-dose oral methotrexate with expectant management of ectopic pregnancy. Obstet Gynecol 1996; 88:775–8.

18. Kirk E, Gevaert O, Haider Z, et al. Can the hCG ratio be used to predict likelihood of success of conservative management of ectopic pregnancies? Ultrasound Obstet Gynecol 2005; 26:362.

10

The medical management of ectopic pregnancy

Emma Kirk

Introduction • Methotrexate • Case report 1 • Case report 2 • Conclusions • Practical points

INTRODUCTION

As discussed in previous chapters, we have seen how high-resolution transvaginal ultrasonography (TVS) and rapid assays of serum human chorionic gonadotrophin (hCG) allow an early diagnosis of pregnancy location to be made in most cases. This has led to more ectopic pregnancies being detected in asymptomatic women. We have heard that in some units over 90% of ectopic pregnancies are visualized on TVS.[1] We know that surgical management is not always appropriate for these women. Both expectant and medical management have been shown to be safe and effective in selected cases of ectopic pregnancy.[2,3] Having already described in the previous chapter how a 'watch and wait' policy can work for some ectopic pregnancies, this chapter aims to give an overview of the use of medical management in the treatment of tubal ectopic pregnancies.

METHOTREXATE

There are reports on the use of RU486, glucose, potassium chloride and actinomycin D in the management of ectopic pregnancies.[4] However, the most commonly used drug is methotrexate, which was first introduced in the 1980s. It is a chemotherapeutic agent that binds to the enzyme dihydrofolate reductase, which is involved in the synthesis of purine nucleotides. It interferes with DNA synthesis and as a consequence disrupts cell multiplication. It can be used both systemically and locally for the treatment of both tubal and non-tubal ectopic pregnancies.

Single-dose methotrexate

Methotrexate is most commonly given systemically according to a single-dose regimen (Table 10.1).[5] In most units this involves giving a dose of $50\,mg/m^2$ on the day of presentation or

---

Table 10.1. Protocol for the use of single dose methotrexate in unruptured ectopic pregnancy

Day	Management
0	Serum hCG, FBC, U&Es, LFTs, G&S
1	Serum hCG
	Intramuscular methotrexate $50\,mg/m^2$
4	Serum hCG
7	Serum hCG, FBC, LFT
	2nd dose of methotrexate if hCG decrease <15% days 4–7
	If hCG decrease >15% repeat hCG weekly until <12 IU/L

Table 10.2. Success rates for single dose methotrexate – a review of the literature. (Reproduced from[29]

Author and reference	Year	N =	Success single dose	Overall success	Additional dose n =	Mean hCG (IU/L)	Time to resolution (days)
Stovall[5]	1993	120	91% (109/120)	94.2% (113/120)	3.3% (4/120)	3950 ± 1193	35.5 ± 11.8
Glock[8]	1994	35	85.7% (30/35)	85.7% (30/35)		1388 ± 464	23.1 ± 2.9
Henry[9]	1994	61	59% (36/61)	85% (52/61)	26.2% (16/61)		
Ransom[10]	1994	21	67% (14/21)	71% (15/21)	4.8% (1/21)	1575 ± 1350	
Corsan[11]	1995	44	52% (23/44)	75% (33/44)	22.7% (10/44)	2517 ± 3144	
Gross[12]	1995	17		94.1% (16/17)		3320 (158–12 420)	26.4 (12–55)
Stika[13]	1997	50	64% (32/50)	78% (39/50)	14% (7/50)	1896.4 ± 2399	26.5 ± 17
Lecuru[14]	1998	37	83.7% (31/37)	91.8% (34/37)	8.1% (3/37)	585 (50–5525)	27.1 (7–50)
Saraj[15]	1998	38	78.9% (30/38)	94.7% (36/38)	15.8% (6/38)	3162 ± 772	27.2 ± 2.3
Gazvani[16]	1998	25	72% (18/25)	88% (22/25)	16% (4/25)		
Thoen[17]	1998	47	76.6% (36/47)	91.5% (43/47)	14.9% (7/47)	803 (45–49 473)	25 ± 15
Elito[18]	1999	40	75% (30/40)	85% (34/40)			
Tawfiq[19]	2000	60	73% (44/60)				25.7 ± 8.8
Sowter[20]	2001	34		65% (22/34)	26% (9/34)		
Lewis-Bliehall[21]	2001	119	70% (83/119)	79% (94/119)	9.2% (11/19)		
Olofsson[22]	2001	26		77% (20/26)			24 ± 9
el-Lamie[23]	2002	35	71% (25/35)	94.3% (33/35)	22.9% (8/35)		34.8 (15–70)
Gamzu[24]	2002	56	89.3% (50/56)			2167 ± 220	
Potter[25]	2003	81		85% (69/81)			
Alshimmiri[26]	2003	77		95% (73/77)		2592 ± 3771	
Erdem[6]	2004	34	65% (22/34)	88% (30/34)	26.6% (8/34)	2490 ± 2912	
Lipscomb[27]	2004	495		90.5% (448/495)			

Comments on inclusion criteria	*Comments*

- Increase in hCG after uterine curettage
- Ectopic mass seen on TVS in 94.2% (113/120)
- Cardiac activity in 11.7% (14/113)
- 17% visualized EP on TVS
- 83% diagnosed after increase in hCG after uterine curettage
- No fetal cardiac activity
- Increase in hCG after uterine curettage
- No fetal cardiac activity

- Diagnosis of ectopic pregnancy based on TVS, hCG and uterine curettage
- Serum hCG <15 000 IU/L
- No fetal cardiac activity

- Serum hCG <5000 IU/L
- 100% success when hCG <3600 IU/L

- Confirmed laparoscopically

- No fetal cardiac activity
- 28% (13/47) visited emergency department because of pain

- USS diagnosis (haematosalpinx, tubal ring or live embryo)

- Ultrasound diagnosis in 70%
- 92.5% success hCG <4000 IU/L
- 35% success hCG >4000 IU/L

- Serum hCG <5000 IU/L

- 48.5% had an adnexal mass 3.6–5.0 cm on TVS

- Ectopic mass seen on TVS in 80% (45/56)
- 5 cases had hCG <1000 IU/L
- Size of ectopic not related to success rate

- Presence of a yolk sac on TVS was a predictor of failure

- Diagnosis on TVS and serial hCG quantification

- No limit on hCG
- Fetal cardiac activity not an exclusion criteria

diagnosis (day 1). Serum hCG levels are then checked on days 4 and 7 post treatment. If the hCG level decreases by more than 15% between days 4 and 7, hCG levels are then checked on a weekly basis. If the hCG does not decrease by more than 15% a second dose can be given. In 3–27% of cases a second dose is needed.[5,6] This protocol has been prospectively validated and been found to identify 90.9% of cases likely to have a successful outcome.[7] Absolute contraindications to its use include significant pain, signs of an acute haemoperitoneum, and liver, kidney or bone marrow impairment. Relative contraindications include fetal cardiac activity, an ectopic mass greater than 3 cm in diameter and an initial hCG level greater than 5000 IU/L. As with expectant management, patient selection is extremely important. Women receiving methotrexate must be reliable and compliant and counselled appropriately before its administration. Although side effects from a single dose of methotrexate are rare, they include nausea, gastric disturbance, tiredness and abdominal pain. Women should be advised to avoid alcohol, folic acid and sexual intercourse during the period of treatment.

Success rates

Reported success rates of single dose methotrexate vary from 65 to 95%.[5,6,8–27] Table 10.2 summarizes published data from 1993–2004 on tubal ectopic pregnancies managed medically with single-dose methotrexate identified using a Medline search.[28] Success rates vary due to different inclusion criteria. Some studies have high success rates due to the inclusion of 'pregnancies of unknown location', not necessarily visualized ectopic pregnancies and women known to have decreasing hCG levels. As shown in the previous chapter these pregnancies may have resolved without any intervention. Other studies with lower success rates include women with fetal cardiac activity, haemoperitoneum and high initial serum hCG levels who may have been excluded from other studies. Lower success rates are seen in the presence of positive fetal cardiac activity.[29] This is probably a reflection of higher hCG levels and more active trophoblast. Both of these have

been associated with decreased success of methotrexate. The presence of a haemoperitoneum could indicate either rupture of the ectopic pregnancy or tubal miscarriage. In the latter one would expect methotrexate to work well as the pregnancy has already failed. This might explain why a recent study showed a success rate of 62% in haemodynamically stable women with suspected ruptured ectopic pregnancy.[30]

In our unit we have managed 56 cases of tubal ectopic pregnancy with single-dose methotrexate. All cases had an ectopic mass visualized on TVS prior to treatment. Inclusion criteria for methotrexate include an hCG of <5000 IU/L, no signs of rupture and an absence of fetal cardiac activity. 44 women received methotrexate as an initial management option with a success rate of 72.7% (32/44). The other 12 women received methotrexate after a period of expectant management with a success rate of 91.7% (11/12). The overall success rate of methotrexate was 76.8% (43/56); 10.7% (6/56) required a second dose.

Predictors of success

The single most important factor in predicting the likely success of methotrexate is probably the initial serum hCG level.[29] Rates of failure have been found to be significantly higher when the initial serum hCG level is greater than 1000 IU/L.[31] The trend in hCG levels before and after methotrexate administration is also an indicator of treatment success and a predictor of possible tubal rupture. If the serum hCG level increases more than 66% over 48 hours before diagnosis and although an initial rise in serum hCG after methotrexate is not unusual, if it persistently rises the threshold for surgical intervention should be lowered.[32] Serum progesterone levels appear to be lower in those treated successfully compared to those who fail treatment with methotrexate, but the difference is not significant.[27] A previous history of ectopic pregnancy is an independent risk factor for the failure of systemic methotrexate.[27] However, the likelihood of failure is not influenced by the method of treatment of the previous ectopic.

Table 10.3. Protocol for the use of multiple dose methotrexate in unruptured ectopic pregnancy

Days	Management
0	Serum hCG, FBC, U&Es, LFTs, G&S
1, 3, 5	Serum hCG
	Intramuscular methotrexate 1 mg/kg
2, 4, 6	Serum hCG
	Intramuscular folinic acid 0.1 mg/kg
	Monitoring
	Continue until hCG decreased >15% in 48 hours or four doses of methotrexate given

Studies have looked at the addition of mifeprostone to increase the efficacy of methotrexate. One randomized study of over 200 ectopic pregnancies failed to demonstrate any benefit except when the serum progesterone was greater than 10 ng/L.[33]

Other methods of administration

Some units favour a multiple-dose regimen for the administration of methotrexate. This involves giving 1 mg/kg on days 1, 3 and 5 with folinic acid rescue on days 2, 4 and 6 (Table 10.3). A review of over 1300 cases of ectopic pregnancy treated either with the single-dose or the multiple-dose regimen found that the multiple-dose regimen was more successful, but associated with significantly more side effects.[34] Methotrexate can also be given orally or intravenously with success rates of 86% and 71% respectively; however there appear to be no obvious advantages over an intramuscular route of administration.[35,36]

Methotrexate can be injected locally at the time of laparoscopy or transvaginally under ultrasound guidance. Direct intra-amniotic injection under ultrasound guidance has proved to be superior to blind intratubal injection at the time of laparoscopy.[37] Studies have shown similar success rates for locally and systemically administered methotrexate.[38] However, systemic administration is preferable, as its administration does not require the same degree of training and skill.

Reproductive outcome

Reproductive outcome after medical management of ectopic pregnancy has been assessed in the form of tubal patency rates on hysterosalpingograms and also subsequent pregnancy rates. Ipsilateral tubal patency rates of 77–82% have been demonstrated on post-treatment hysterosalpingograms in cases treated with single-dose systemic methotrexate.[5,8,39] These rates are comparable to those seen after linear salpingostomy.[39] Subsequent pregnancy rates of over 80% have been reported.[5,40] A total of 82–87% of these were intrauterine and 13–18% ectopic pregnancies. One study showed that the mean time to achieve pregnancy was 3.2 ± 1.1 months from the time of treatment.[5] A previous history of infertility appears to be an important factor associated with a poor reproductive performance.[40]

Comparison to surgery

Single- and multiple-dose methotrexate regimens have been compared to surgical treatment. No significant differences were found in primary treatment success or tubal preservation in a randomized trial involving women with a laparoscopically confirmed tubal ectopic pregnancy following either multiple-dose systemic methotrexate or laparoscopic salpingotomy.[41] Three randomized studies have shown that single-dose methotrexate is significantly less effective than laparoscopic salpingotomy.[15,20,42] Although women treated with methotrexate had significantly better objective physical functioning scores there were no differences in any other psychological outcomes.[20]

Various economic comparisons have been made between the use of methotrexate and surgery. In The Netherlands it has been shown that systemic methotrexate therapy can reduce costs if administered to patients with low initial serum hCG levels without confirmatory laparoscopy.[42] Similarly in New Zealand it has been shown that single-dose methotrexate resulted in a 52% reduction in direct costs and a 40% reduction in indirect costs compared to laparoscopic surgery.[44] Women with hCG levels of >1500 IU/L had higher indirect costs due to an increased likelihood of surgical intervention and prolonged follow up.

SUGGESTED MANAGEMENT PROTOCOL

Units offering conservative management of ectopic pregnancies should have clear protocols including details of inclusion and exclusion criteria and the follow up needed. It is also essential that women undergoing such management have access 24 hours a day to healthcare professionals if any problems arise. For example, in our unit patients have direct access to one of the medical staff at all times, by mobile phone, for advice.

After an ectopic pregnancy has been diagnosed and ultrasonographic criteria for medical management have been fulfilled, such as the absence of fetal cardiac activity and haemoperitoneum, as with expectant management a bimanual vaginal examination should be performed. Provided there is no cervical excitation or adnexal tenderness and the woman is haemodynamically stable, blood should be sent for full blood count, urea and electrolytes, liver function tests, hCG, progesterone and group and save. If these are normal and the hCG level is below the cut-off level used in a particular unit for medical management, methotrexate may be given. A single dose of methotrexate should be given at a dose of 50 mg/m.[2] Follow up should be in accordance with Stovall's original protocol as detailed above. In our unit we adopt a variation of this protocol and advocate repeating the hCG at 48 hours before deciding to give methotrexate, enabling the pretreatment hCG ratio (hCG 48 h/hCG 0 h) to be calculated. This will avoid the need to unnecessarily administer methotrexate to women with spontaneously failing ectopic pregnancies, i.e. those with an hCG ratio of <0.8, who are likely to have successful expectant management.[45] This pretreatment hCG ratio can also be used to predict the likely success from methotrexate treatment. If the hCG ratio is less than 1.6, there is almost an 80% chance of success with

methotrexate.[45] As the hCG ratio increases the chances of successful medical management decrease accordingly. The majority of women treated with methotrexate can be safely managed as outpatients. If the woman develops any pain she should undergo repeat bimanual and TVS examinations and blood tests. Abdominal pain is a common side effect of methotrexate and often admission for a short time until this settles is all that is required; however, it is important to realize when managing ectopic pregnancies conservatively that rupture can occur and the patient must be told explicitly that this is a risk and that she must contact the hospital if she has concerns. All women who complain of pain must be assessed to exclude tubal rupture and in some cases a laparoscopy and definitive surgical treatment will be indicated.

All rhesus-negative women with an ectopic pregnancy treated conservatively should also receive anti-D immunoglobulin.

Figure 10.1 suggests a protocol for the conservative management of ectopic pregnancy.

The following two cases illustrate the spectrum of outcomes when methotrexate is used for the management of ectopic pregnancy.

CASE REPORT 1

A 33-year-old woman presented to the EPU for a dating scan, as she was unsure of her last menstrual period. She had had some light vaginal spotting over the previous 3 days but no associated pain. A TVS was performed. The uterine cavity appeared empty but there was a 16 × 17 × 16 mm right adnexal mass with a visible gestational sac ('bagel sign') (see Figure 10.2). She was given the diagnosis of a right tubal ectopic pregnancy. Blood was taken. The initial hCG was 208 IU/L and progesterone 6 nmol/L. As she was asymptomatic she was offered a repeat hCG in 48 hours to see if she could be managed expectantly. However as it was an unplanned pregnancy she was keen to undergo immediate treatment so received 75 mg methotrexate (50 mg/m²). Serum hCG levels were repeated on days 4 and 7. They were 225 IU/L and 165 IU/L respectively. The hCG had decreased by 27% between days 4 and

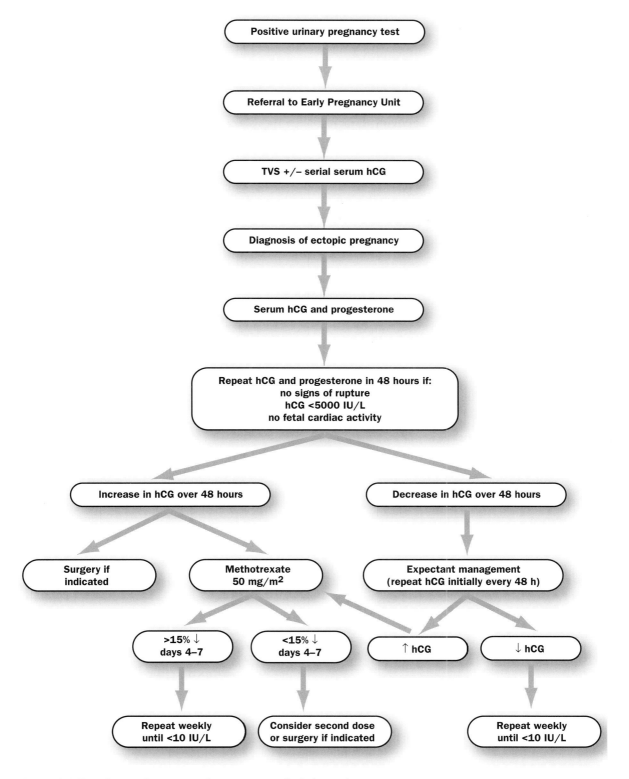

Figure 10.1 Flow diagram for suggested management of tubal ectopic pregnancy

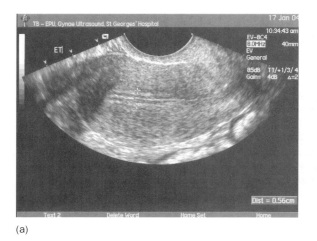
(a)

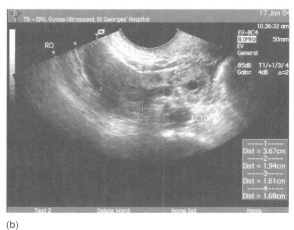
(b)

Figure 10.2 Transvaginal scan images showing (a) an empty uterine cavity and (b) a right ectopic pregnancy ('bagel sign')

7 so the decision was made to repeat the hCG in 1 week. Unfortunately she developed pain on day 8 post-methotrexate and so returned to the EPU. A repeat TVS showed evidence of a haemoperitoneum and as she was in pain, the decision was made to perform a laparoscopy. At laparoscopy she was found to have 200 ml haemoperitoneum and a ruptured right ectopic pregnancy. A salpingectomy was performed and she made a good postoperative recovery.

Notes

- Ectopic pregnancies can still rupture even when the hCG has decreased.
- It is essential that women be in contact with the EPU until hCG levels have returned to normal.

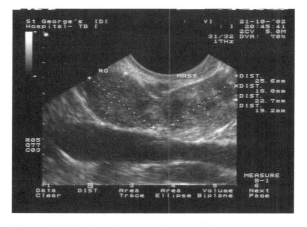

Figure 10.3 Transvaginal scan images showing an inhomogeneous mass next to the right ovary

CASE REPORT 2

A 25-year-old woman was referred to the EPU from the Accident and Emergency Department. She attended with a 2-day history of light vaginal bleeding. It was her first pregnancy and she was 6^{+3} weeks according to her last menstrual period. A transvaginal scan was performed which showed an empty uterus and an inhomogeneous mass in the right adnexa (see Figure 10.3). The serum hCG was 1739 IU/L and the progesterone 9 nmol/L. As she was relatively asymptomatic and had minimal tenderness on examination the hormone levels were repeated in 48 hours. At 48 hours the hCG was 1692 IU/L and the progesterone was 8 nmol/l. The decision was therefore to manage expectantly. A further hCG level, now 96 hours from diagnosis was 1702 IU/L and the progesterone 8 nmol/L. As the hCG had plateaued a single dose of methotrexate was given at a dose

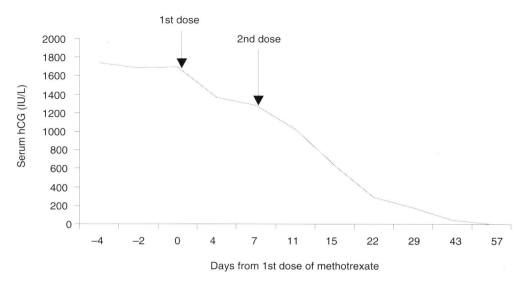

Figure 10.4 Graph to show a typical pattern of hCG decrease after systemic methotrexate

of 50 mg/m^2. The hCG decreased only 6% between days 4 and 7, with levels of 1423 IU/L and 1285 IU/L respectively. Therefore a second dose of 50 mg/m^2 was given. With the second dose there was a decrease in hCG of 29% between days 4 and 7. Levels were then monitored on a weekly basis. Within 8 weeks of diagnosis the hCG was less than 10 IU/L (Figure 10.4). A repeat TVS 3 months post-treatment showed no obvious residual ectopic mass.

Notes

- Up to 25% of women may need a second dose of methotrexate.
- Methotrexate can still be successful if administration is delayed by a period of initial expectant management immediately after diagnosis.

CONCLUSIONS

Medical management of tubal ectopic pregnancies should be offered to selected women who are clinically stable with a serum hCG level of <5000 IU/L. If the hCG ratio is used then a pretreatment ratio of 1.6 is associated with optimal results. These women can be managed as outpatients, but close follow up with after-hours support is essential if women are to be treated with more conservative approaches. The most appropriate and easiest regimen is a single dose of methotrexate (50 mg/m^2) and currently successful management correlates well with a fall in the level of serum hCG of more than 15% between days 4 and 7. One would expect high rates of ipsilateral tubal patency after methotrexate treatment. It is important to remember that an ectopic pregnancy can rupture even in the presence of falling serum hCG levels.

PRACTICAL POINTS

1. Methotrexate is safe and effective for the management of tubal ectopic pregnancy.
2. Appropriate case selection is important.
3. Any women managed medically should be able to have contact with a healthcare professional 24 hours a day.
4. Success rates are higher if the initial serum hCG level is less than 2000 IU/L.

REFERENCES

1. Condous G, Okaro E, Khalid A, et al. The accuracy of transvaginal ultrasonography for the diagnosis of ectopic pregnancy prior to surgery. Hum Reprod 2005; 20:1404–9.

2. Korhonen J, Stenman UH, Ylostalo P. Serum human chorionic gonadotrophin dynamics during spontaneous resolution of ectopic pregnancy. Fertil Steril 1994; 61:632–6.

3. Parker J, Bisits A, Proietto AM. A systematic review of single-dose intramuscular methotrexate for the treatment of ectopic pregnancy. Aust NZ J Obstet Gynecol 1998; 38:145–50.

4. Kooi S, Kock HC. A review of the literature on nonsurgical treatment in tubal pregnancies. Obstet Gynecol Surv 1992; 47:739–49.

5. Stovall TG, Ling FW. Single dose methotrexate: an expanded clinical trial. Am J Obstet Gynecol 1993; 168:1759–65.

6. Erdem M, Erdem A, Arslan M, et al. Single dose methotrexate for the treatment of unruptured ectopic pregnancy. Arch Gynecol Obstet 2004; 270:201–4.

7. Kirk E, Condous G, Van Calster B, Haider Z, Bourne T. Is it possible to predict successful treatment response to methotrexate earlier than seven days? Ultrasound Obstet Gynecol 2005; 26:456.

8. Glock JL, Johnson JV, Brumsted JR. Efficacy and safety of single-dose methotrexate in the treatment of ectopic pregnancy. Fertil Steril 1994; 62:716–21.

9. Henry MA, Gentry WL. Single injection of methotrexate for treatment of ectopic pregnancies. Am J Obstet Gynecol 1994; 171:1584–7.

10. Ransom MX, Garcia AJ, Bohrer M, Corsan GH, Kemmann E. Serum progesterone as a predictor of success in the treatment of ectopic pregnancy. Obstet Gynaecol 1994; 83:1033–7.

11. Corsan GH, Karacan M, Qasim S, et al. Identification of hormonal parameters for successful systemic single-dose methotrexate therapy in ectopic pregnancy. Hum Reprod 1995; 10:2719–22.

12. Gross Z, Rodriguez JJ, Stalnaker BL. Ectopic pregnancy. Nonsurgical, outpatient evaluation and single-dose methotrexate treatment. J Reprod Med 1995; 40:371–4.

13. Stika CS, Anderson L, Frederiksen MC. Single-dose methotrexate for the treatment of ectopic pregnancy: Northwestern Memorial Hospital three-year experience. Am J Obstet Gynecol 1996; 174:1840–6.

14. Lecuru F, Robin F, Bernard JP, et al. Single-dose methotrexate for unruptured ectopic pregnancy. Int J Gynaecol Obstet 1998; 61:253–9.

15. Saraj AJ, Wilcox JG, Najmabadi S, et al. Resolution of hormonal markers of ectopic gestation: a randomized trial comparing single-dose intramuscular methotrexate with salpingostomy. Obstet Gynecol 1998; 92:989–94.

16. Gazvani MR, Baruah DN, Alfirevic Z, Emery SJ. Mifeprostone in combination with methotrexate for the medical treatment of tubal pregnancy: a randomized, controlled trial. Hum Reprod 1998; 13:1987–90.

17. Thoen LD, Creinin MD. Medical treatment of ectopic pregnancy with methotrexate. Fertil Steril 1997; 68:727–30.

18. Elito J Jr, Reichmann AP, Uchiyama MN, Camano L. Predictive score for the systemic treatment of unruptured ectopic pregnancy with a single dose of methotrexate. Int J Gynaecol Obstet 1999; 67:75–9.

19. Tawfiq A, Agameya AF, Claman P. Predictors of treatment failure for ectopic pregnancy treated with single-dose methotrexate. Fertil Steril 2000; 74:877–80.

20. Sowter MC, Farquhar CM, Petrie KJ, Gudex G. A randomized trial comparing single dose systemic methotrexate and laparoscopic surgery for the treatment of unruptured tubal pregnancy. BJOG 2001; 108:192–203.

21. Lewis-Bliehall C, Rogers RG, Kammerer-Doak DN, et al. Medical vs. surgical treatment of ectopic pregnancy. The university of New Mexico's six-year experience. J Reprod Med 2001; 46:983–8.

22. Olofsson JI, Poromaa IS, Ottander U, Kjellberg L, Damber MG. Clinical and pregnancy outcome following ectopic pregnancy; a prospective study comparing expectancy, surgery and systemic methotrexate treatment. Acta Obstet Gynecol Scand 2001; 80:744–9.

23. el-Lamie IK, Shehata NA, Kamel HA. Intramuscular methotrexate for tubal pregnancy. J Reprod Med 2002; 47:144–50.

24. Gamzu R, Almog B, Levin Y, et al. The ultrasonographic appearance of tubal pregnancy in patients treated with methotrexate. Hum Reprod 2002; 17:2585–7.

25. Potter MB, Lepine LA, Jamieson DJ. Predictors of success with methotrexate treatment of tubal ectopic pregnancy at Grady Memorial Hospital. Am J Obstet Gynecol 2003; 188:1192–94.

26. Alshimmiri MM, Al-Saleh EA, Al-Harmi JA, et al. Treatment of ectopic pregnancy with a single intramuscular dose of methotrexate. Arch Gynecol Obstet 2003; 268:181–3.

27. Lipscomb GH, Givens VA, Meyer NL, Bran D. Previous ectopic pregnancy as a predictor of failure of systemic methotrexate therapy. Fertil Steril 2004; 81:1221–4.

28. Lipscomb GH, McCord ML, Stovall TG, et al. Predictors of success of methotrexate treatment in women with ectopic pregnancies. N Engl J Med 1999; 341:1974–8.

29. Kirk E, Condous G, Bourne T. The non-surgical management of ectopic pregnancy. Ultrasound Obstet Gynecol 2006; 27:91–100.

30. Kumtepe Y, Kadanali S. Medical treatment of ruptured with haemodynamically stable and unruptured ectopic pregnancy patients. Eur J Obstet Gynecol Reprod Biol 2004; 116:221–225.

31. Nazac A, Gervaise A, Bouyer J, et al. Predictors of success in methotrexate treatment of women with unruptured tubal pregnancies. Ultrasound Obstet Gynecol 2003; 21:181–5.

32. Dudley PS, Heard MJ, Sangi-Haghpeykar H, Carson SA, Buster JE. Characterizing ectopic pregnancies that rupture despite treatment with methotrexate. Fertil Steril 2004; 82:1374–8.

33. Rozenberg P, Chevret S, Camus E, et al. Medical treatment of ectopic pregnancies: a randomized clinical trial comparing methotrexate-mifeprostone and methotrexate-placebo. Hum Reprod 2003; 18:1802–8.

34. Barnhart KT, Gosman G, Ashby R, Sammel M. The medical management of ectopic pregnancy: a meta-analysis comparing 'single dose' and 'multidose' regimens. Obstet Gynecol 2003; 101:778–84.

35. Lipscomb GH, Meyer NL, Flynn DE, Peterson M, Ling FW. Oral methotrexate for treatment of ectopic pregnancy. Am J Obstet Gynecol 2002; 186:1192–1195.

36. Pentil 2004 Periti E, Comparetto C, Villanucci A, Coccia ME, Tavella K, Amunni G. The use of intravenous methotrexate in the treatment of ectopic pregnancy. J Chemother 2004; 16:211–15.

37. Tzafettas J, Anapliotis S, Zournatzi V, et al. Transvaginal intra-amniotic injection of methotrexate in early ectopic pregnancy. Advantages over the laparoscopic approach. Early Hum Dev 1994; 39:101–7.

38. Fernandez H, Benifla JL, Lelaidier C, Baton C, Frydman R. Methotrexate treatment of ectopic pregnancy: 100 cases treated by primary transvaginal injection under sonographic control. Fertil Steril 1993; 59:773–7.

39. Tolaymat LL, Brown TL, Maher JE, et al. Reproductive potential after methotrexate treatment of ectopic gestation in a community hospital. J Reprod Med 1999; 44:335–8.

40. Gervaise A, Mason L, de Tayrac R, Frydman R, Fernandez H. Reproductive outcome after methotrexate treatment of tubal pregnancies. Fertil Steril 2004; 82: 304–8.

41. Hajenius PJ, Engelsbel S, Mol BW, et al. Randomised trial of systemic methotrexate versus laparoscopic salpingostomy in tubal pregnancy. Lancet 1997; 350:774–9.

42. Fernandez H, Yves Vincent SC, Pauthier S, Audibert F, Frydman R. Randomized trial of conservative laparoscopic treatment and methotrexate administration in ectopic pregnancy and subsequent fertility. Hum Reprod 1998; 13:3239–43.

43. Mol BW, Hajenius PJ, Engelsbel S, et al. Treatment of tubal pregnancy in The Netherlands: an economic comparison of systemic methotrexate administration and laparoscopic salpingostomy. Am J Obstet Gynecol 1999; 181:945–51.

44. Sowter MC, Farquhar CM, Gudex G. An economic evaluation of single dose systemic methotrexate and laparoscopic surgery for the treatment of unruptured ectopic pregnancy. BJOG 2001; 108:204–12.

45. Kirk E, Gevaert O, Haider Z, Condous G, Bourne T. Can the hCG ratio be used to predict likelihood of success of conservative management of ectopic pregnancies? Ultrasound Obstet Gynecol 2005; 26:362.

11

The surgical treatment of ectopic pregnancy

Olav Istre

Introduction • Surgical treatment • Laparoscopy versus laparotomy • Linear salpingotomy versus salpingectomy • Surgical treatment of non-tubal ectopic pregnancy • Conclusions • Practical points

INTRODUCTION

The increased incidence of ectopic pregnancy seen over recent decades has occurred simultaneously with an increased incidence of pelvic inflammatory disease. This suggests a causal relationship (Figure 11.1). Improvements in the treatment of pelvic inflammatory diseases may now preserve tubal function in women who previously would have suffered from tubal factor infertility. However, more recently in Norway a fall in the incidence of ectopic pregnancy has been reported.[1] It has been suggested that the falling rates of pelvic inflam-

matory disease may be responsible for these changes.

Ectopic pregnancy can be defined as the implantation of a fertilized ovum anywhere other than in the endometrial cavity. Ninety-five per cent of ectopic pregnancies occur within the fallopian tube (Table 11.1). Non-tubal ectopic pregnancies, including caesarean section scar pregnancy are discussed elsewhere in this book.[2,3]

It can be argued that the use of transvaginal ultrasonography (Figure 11.2) and the treatment of ectopic pregnancy using minimal access surgery has contributed to the decreased

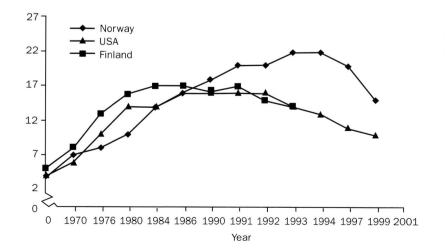

Figure 11.1 Ectopic pregnancy trends (from Sintef Health)

Table 11.1. Localization of ectopic pregnancy	
Fallopian tube	
• Ampullary segment	80%
• Isthmic segment	10%
• Fimbrial end	5%
• Cornual and interstitial	2%
Abdominal	1.4%
Ovarian	0.2%
Cervical	0.2%

Table 11.2. History of the treatment of ectopic pregnancy

- 1876 expectant management mortality rate 69% (Parry, Philadelphia)
- First salpingectomy by Lawson Tait (1884)
- First salpingotomy by Stromme
  - Obstet Gynecol 1953;1:427–9
- Laparoscopic salpingectomy:
  - Shapiro & Adler Am J Obstet Gynecol 1973:117:290–1
- Laparoscopic salpingotomy:
  - Bruhat, Manhes, Choukroun, Suzanne Francaise de Gynecologie et d'Obstetrique 1977;72:667–9.

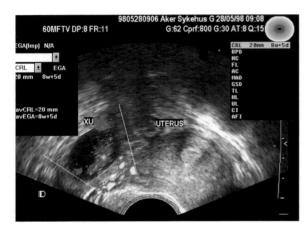

Figure 11.2 Transvaginal ultrasound of a live ectopic pregnancy at 8 weeks 5 days. (See also colour plate)

mortality rate associated with this condition. The result is that the management of unruptured tubal pregnancy has changed from being focused on immediate, life-saving intervention to making more effort to preserve fertility. The treatment options that are available for a given ectopic pregnancy relate to the location, with the majority of tubal ectopic pregnancies surgical management is safe and effective. This chapter will focus on the surgical approach to the management of this condition.

SURGICAL TREATMENT

Preservation of the fallopian tube containing an extrauterine pregnancy may maintain fertility. This approach was first described in the German literature by Prochownic in 1894. He performed a 'salpingotomi' operation which was followed 2 years later in the same woman by a successful pregnancy.[4] By 1952 there were still few reports in the literature reporting the use of salpingotomy for tubal pregnancy (Table 11.2); however, a case report that year described a woman with an ectopic pregnancy in her remaining tube which underwent surgical treatment. Following this the women had two subsequent intrauterine pregnancies.[5,6]

In 1967 Timonen put forward the view that radical surgical treatment is not justified in childless women when the contralateral tube is severely damaged.[7] The value of laparoscopy as a diagnostic procedure was emphasized by Hope more than 50 years ago.[8] In order to assess its value, a study was made on 489 laparoscopies performed for suspected ectopic pregnancy. The total diagnostic accuracy was 98.5%.[9] The laparoscope remained a purely diagnostic tool, until in 1973 Shapiro reported the first operative laparoscopy for ectopic pregnancy. More recently the use of vaginal ultrasonography and serum hCG levels has made the laparoscope almost redundant as a diagnostic tool. However it has come to the fore for treatment. The appropriate surgical technique when operating on ectopic pregnancies depends not only on the location of the ectopic gestation and the extent of tubal damage that results, but also on the woman's future wishes, the technical expertise of the surgeon, and the equipment available.[10] Throughout the 1980s, the use of the laparoscope for surgery was developed until it became standard for the management for ectopic pregnancy; however, the debate over the relative merits of laparoscopic and open surgery did not resolve easily.

LAPAROSCOPY VERSUS LAPAROTOMY

The first laparoscopic treatment of this condition was reported in 1973 by Shapiro.[11] Although several series have since been published,[12] the technique took some time to gain general acceptance. There were predictable surgical complications and significant problems with training.

There were initial concerns about tubal patency and adhesion formation after laparoscopic treatment versus traditional laparotomy for ectopic pregnancy. However more recently these concerns have been resolved. Virtually all studies have shown that laparoscopic surgery is superior to laparotomy. Lower cost, shorter hospital stay, less operative time, less blood loss, reduced analgesia requirements and shorter convalescence have been demonstrated in the laparoscopic group.[13] Table 11.3 shows the rates of subsequent intrauterine pregnancy were 62% after laparotomy and 59% after laparoscopy, and the rates of ectopic pregnancies were 16% and 12% respectively. These data suggest that there are no significant differences in reproductive outcome following laparoscopy or laparotomy. The issue of adhesion formation was addressed by Fayad et al. Two groups were investigated in this study,[14] 396 women had a laparotomy, and 546 women underwent operative laparoscopy. This study concluded that there was no therapeutic advantage to the use of Ringers solution (instilled into the abdominal cavity) for the prevention of postoperative pelvic adhesion formation, but in the laparoscopy group no adhesions developed in women who had pelviolysis or fimbrioplasty.[14]

Despite the fact that women with a tubal pregnancy in their only fallopian tube are a very high-risk group, it is possible to restore

Table 11.3. Outcome after laparoscopy or laparotomy treatment of ectopic pregnancy				
Authors	Year	No	% IUP	% EP
DeCherney	1987	69	52	16
Donnez	1990	138	51	10
Pouly	1990	223	67	12
Paulsen	1992	48	54	31
Total laparoscopy		478	59	12
Timonen	1967	185	53	12
Sherman	1982	47	83	6
Querleu	1988	129	52	30
Tuomivaara	1988	86	66	14
Makinen	1989	42	69	29
Langer	1990	118	70	11
Total laparotomy		607	62	16

tubal function in a high proportion of cases. In one report 16 of 21 women who subsequently conceived were treated with laparotomy and microsurgery to the remaining fallopian tube.[15]

However, tubal function following an ectopic pregnancy is a significant problem as there may be pre-existing pathology. Approximately 50% of 76 women with a history of previous pelvic inflammatory disease and a laparotomy for ectopic pregnancy were found to have a non-patent contralateral tube on follow up hysterosalpingography. In the same study a subgroup of 13 women were managed by linear salpingotomy. In only six cases was the treated tube subsequently found to be patent.[16]

The laparoscopic approach for the treatment of ectopic pregnancy is believed to be associated with improved fertility – perhaps because of reduced adhesion formation. In one study, 105 women with ectopic pregnancy were randomized to laparoscopy or laparotomy. Women who underwent a laparotomy developed significantly more adhesions than women who underwent a laparoscopy.[17] In a further three studies which compared laparoscopy and laparotomy for the treatment of ectopic pregnancy, all concluded that if surgery was performed, the laparoscopic approach should be used.[18,19]

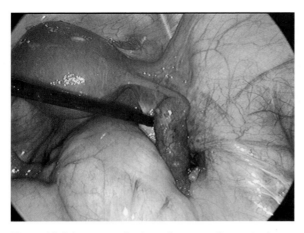

Figure 11.3 Laparoscopic view of an ampullary ectopic pregnancy. (See also colour plate)

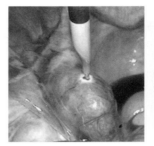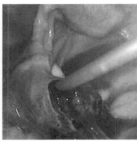

Figure 11.4 Laparoscopic salpingotomy in a left-sided ampullary ectopic pregnancy. (See also colour plate)

LINEAR SALPINGOTOMY VERSUS SALPINGECTOMY

In women who wish to preserve their fertility, conservative surgery by linear salpingotomy is considered the gold standard for the management of ectopic pregnancy (Figure 11.3). In practice, any haemoperitoneum if present is evacuated, the ectopic pregnancy is identified and the tube is immobilized. A 1.5–2.5 cm longitudinal incision is made on the maximally distended ante-mesosalpinx wall of the tube, with a unipolar needle. The products of conception are then flushed out using a suction irrigation device with sterile saline (aquadissection). Gentle blunt dissection may also be necessary. The products of conception can then usually be removed using an endobag, or if this is not available forceps via one of the port sites. Any bleeding points can be coagulated with bipolar diathermy. If bleeding is persistent then laparoscopic suturing may be required. Many surgeons advocate the use of a vasopressin injection into the mesosalpinx prior to any incision in order to reduce the likelihood of bleeding.[20]

So, when is a salpingectomy indicated? Generally in women with tubal rupture, uncontrollable bleeding and when future pregnancies are not desired. Other indications include women who have become pregnant following tubal sterilization and in women who are undergoing IVF treatment.

Despite conservative surgical approaches, future fertility is preserved in only 40–60% of women and there is an increased risk of a further ectopic pregnancy. In the past decade, a number of investigators have reported treatment of tubal pregnancy with salpingotomy as well as medical treatment.

In 266 women who were actively attempting to conceive, salpingectomy or salpingotomy were performed for their first ectopic pregnancy between January 1992 and January 1999. These women were followed for a minimum of 18 months.[21] The cumulative intrauterine pregnancy rate was significantly higher after salpingotomy (88%) than after salpingectomy (66%). No difference was found in the recurrence rate of ectopic pregnancy between the treatments (16% vs 17%). In cases of contralateral tubal pathology, the chance of a future pregnancy was relatively low (hazard ratio 0.463) and the risk of recurrence was high (hazard ratio 2.25). From these data it seems reasonable to conclude that conservative surgery is superior to radical surgery at preserving fertility, although the presence or absence of pathology in the contralateral tube is probably the most important factor.

Management in the presence of contralateral tubal pathology is disputed and should ideally be addressed in a randomized clinical trial. However, a history of previous subfertility is associated with a decreased fertility rate after surgical management of ectopic pregnancy.[22] The recommendation is in vitro fertilization (IVF) to women with a damaged or absent contralateral tube.

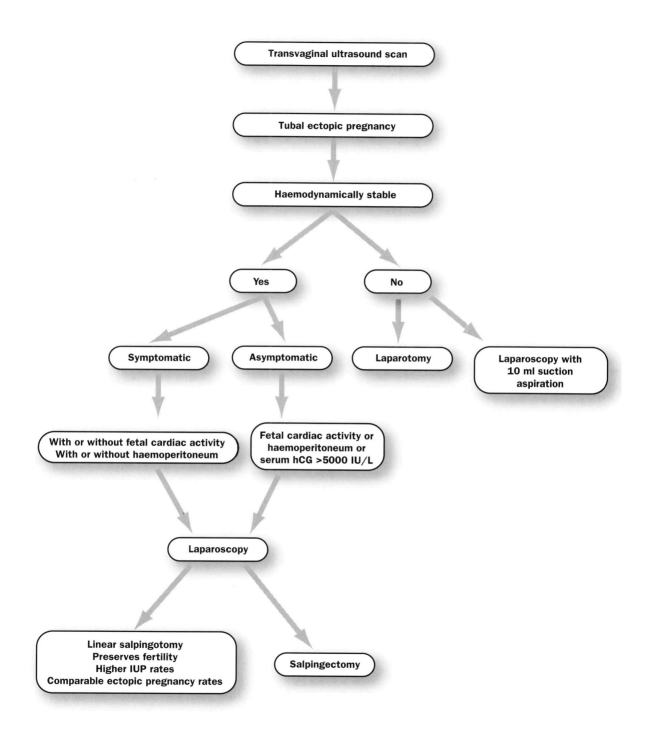

Figure 11.5 Flow diagram to illustrate a surgical management plan for women with an ectopic pregnancy.

Conservative surgery is not followed by an increased risk of repeat ectopic pregnancy, however there is a risk of incomplete removal of functional trophoblast tissue; and persistent trophoblastic tissue has been reported to be as high as 4%.[23] This should be taken into account when deciding on the operative procedure. It is therefore necessary to identify women with persistent disease by monitoring the postoperative serum human chorionic gonadotrophin (hCG) levels.[24] Many authors recommend weekly serum hCG after salpingotomy. However a protocol based on measuring serum hCG on the first postoperative day has also been advocated with a decrease of <50% of the preoperative value being thought to predict persistent ectopic pregnancy.[25]

SURGICAL TREATMENT OF NON-TUBAL ECTOPIC PREGNANCY

Interstitial pregnancy

This is a rare condition (Table 11.1) occurring in 1 per 2500 live births. Women are often asymptomatic until acute haemorrhage occurs late in the first trimester or early second trimester secondary to uterine rupture. The surgical treatment is cornual resection, however if early ultrasound examination confirms the diagnosis, laparoscopic cornual resection is possible[26] with laparoscopic suturing and bipolar coagulation. The injection of potassium chloride or methotrexate has also been reported.[27] In general a surgical approach to these pregnancies is not advised as medical management is usually successful. This is discussed in more detail in Chapter 12.

Abdominal pregnancy

Most abdominal pregnancies are of a secondary type (early tubal abortion or rupture). They represent 1% of ectopic pregnancies and are associated with an eight times higher maternal mortality compared to other ectopic pregnancies and a perinatal mortality of 80–91%. Fetal position is often abnormal and the cervix is displaced and unaffected. The treatment is surgical. Once the pregnancy has been removed the placenta should be left in situ and the active trophoblast that remains treated with methotrexate. This condition should be terminated as soon as the diagnosis is established. In the event of an early diagnosis, this condition can be treated successfully with the laparoscope, if the implantation does not involve a vascular area that may lead to uncontrolled bleeding.

Ovarian pregnancy

This is also a rare condition and accounts for about 1% of the ectopic pregnancies. Laparoscopy establishes both the diagnosis and is the treatment of choice. Removal of the ectopic pregnancy, ovarian wedge resection or oophorectomy can be performed.[28]

PRACTICAL POINTS

1. Ninety-five per cent of ectopic gestations occur within the fallopian tube.
2. The laparoscopic approach in stable women with ectopic pregnancy is superior to the laparotomic.
3. Linear salpingotomy is considered the gold standard for the management of ectopic pregnancy in women who wish to preserve their fertility.
4. The cumulative intrauterine pregnancy rate is significantly higher after linear salpingotomy compared to salpingectomy.
5. There is no signficant difference in the extrauterine pregnancy rate when comparing linear salpingotomy to salpingectomy.
6. Conservative surgery is superior to radical surgery at preserving fertility.
7. Conservative surgery however carries a higher risk of persistent trophoblastic disease.

CONCLUSIONS

If surgery is performed, the treatment of choice for ectopic pregnancy in women who wish to preserve their fertility is laparoscopic salpingotomy (Figure 11.4). The reproductive performance after this operation seems to be better than salpingectomy. The laparoscopic approach has less of a role as a diagnostic tool. Chapter 8 argues that the majority of ectopic pregnancies should be visualized using transvaginal ultrasound prior to surgery. The main role for laparoscopy in the modern management of selected cases of ectopic pregnancy is a therapeutic one. Laparoscopy should be undertaken in a unit with endoscopically trained surgeons; particularly when suturing techniques are mandatory in the more rare types of ectopic pregnancy (Figure 11.5).

REFERENCES

1. Bakken IJ, Skjeldestad FE. Incidence and treatment of extrauterine pregnancies in Norway 1990–2001]. Tidsskr Nor Laegeforen 2003; 123:3016–20.
2. Jurkovic D, Hillaby K, Woelfer B, et al. Cesarean scar pregnancy. Ultrasound Obstet Gynecol 2003; 21:310.
3. Jurkovic D, Hillaby K, Woelfer B, et al. First-trimester diagnosis and management of pregnancies implanted into the lower uterine segment Cesarean section scar. Ultrasound Obstet Gynecol 2003; 21:220–7.
4. Prochownic L. Ein betrage zur mechanic des tubenaborts. Festschr d Gesellsch f Geburts u Gynecil in Berlin. Wien 1884; 266.
5. Stromme WB. Conservative surgery for ectopic pregnancy. A twenty-year review. Obstet Gynecol 1973; 41:215–23.
6. Stromme WB. Salpingotomy for tubal pregnancy; report of a successful case. Obstet Gynecol 1953; 1:472–75.
7. Timonen S, Nieminen U. Tubal pregnancy, choice of operative method of treatment. Acta Obstet Gynecol Scand 1967; 46:327–39.
8. Hope R. Differential diagnosis of ectopic gestation by peritoneoscopy. Surg Gynecol Obstet 1937; 64.
9. Samuelsson S, Sjovall A. Laparoscopy in suspected ectopic pregnancy. Acta Obstet Gynecol Scand 1972; 51:31–5.
10. Diamond MP, DeCherney AH. Surgical techniques in the management of ectopic pregnancy. Clin Obstet Gynecol 1987; 30:200–9.
11. Shapiro HI, Adler DH. Excision of an ectopic pregnancy through the laparoscope. Am J Obstet Gynecol 1973; 117:290–1.
12. Bruhat MA, Manhes H, Mage G, Pouly JL. Treatment of ectopic pregnancy by means of laparoscopy. Fertil Steril 1980; 33:411–14.
13. Yao M, Tulandi T. Current status of surgical and nonsurgical management of ectopic pregnancy. Fertil Steril 1997; 67:421–33.
14. Fayez JA, Schneider PJ. Prevention of pelvic adhesion formation by different modalities of treatment. Am J Obstet Gynecol 1987; 157:1184–8.
15. Oelsner G, Rabinovitch O, Morad J, Mashiach S, Serr DM. Reproductive outcome after microsurgical treatment of tubal pregnancy in women with a single fallopian tube. J Reprod Med 1986; 31:483–6.
16. Mitchell DE, McSwain HF, McCarthy JA, Peterson HB. Hysterosalpingographic evaluation of tubal patency after ectopic pregnancy. Am J Obstet Gynecol 1987; 157:618–22.
17. Lundorff P, Hahlin M, Kallfelt B, Thorburn J, Lindblom B. Adhesion formation after laparoscopic surgery in tubal pregnancy: a randomized trial versus laparotomy. Fertil Steril 1991; 55:911–15.
18. Lundorff P, Thorburn J, Hahlin M, Kallfelt B, Lindblom B. Laparoscopic surgery in ectopic pregnancy. A randomized trial versus laparotomy. Acta Obstet Gynecol Scand 1991; 70:343–48.
19. Baumann R, Magos AL, Turnbull A. Prospective comparison of videopelviscopy with laparotomy for ectopic pregnancy. Br J Obstet Gynaecol 1991; 98:765–71.
20. Ugur M, Yesilyurt H, Soysal S, Gokmen O. Prophylactic vasopressin during laparoscopic salpingotomy for ectopic pregnancy. J Am Assoc Gynecol Laparosc 1996; 3:365–8.
21. Bangsgaard N, Lund CO, Ottesen B, Nilas L. Improved fertility following conservative surgical treatment of ectopic pregnancy. BJOG 2003; 110:765–70.
22. dela CA, Cumming DC. Factors determining fertility after conservative or radical surgical treatment for ectopic pregnancy. Fertil Steril 1997; 68:871–4.
23. Maymon R, Shulman A, Halperin R, Michell A, Bukovsky I. Ectopic pregnancy and laparoscopy: review of 1197 patients treated by salpingectomy or salpingotomy. Eur J Obstet Gynecol Reprod Biol 1995; 62:61–7.
24. Johnson TR Jr, Sanborn JR, Wagner KS, Compton AA. Gonadotropin surveillance following conservative surgery for ectopic pregnancy. Fertil Steril 1980; 33:207–8.
25. Spandorfer SD, Sawin SW, Benjamin I, Barnhart KT. Postoperative day 1 serum human chorionic gonadotropin level as a predictor of persistent ectopic pregnancy after conservative surgical management. Fertil Steril 1997; 68:430–4.

26. Tulandi T, Vilos G, Gomel V. Laparoscopic treatment of interstitial pregnancy. Obstet Gynecol 1995; 85:465–7.

27. Fernandez H, De Ziegler D, Bourget P, Feltain P, Frydman R. The place of methotrexate in the management of interstitial pregnancy. Hum Reprod 1991; 6:302–6.

28. Raziel A, Schachter M, Mordechai E, et al. Ovarian pregnancy – a 12-year experience of 19 cases in one institution. Eur J Obstet Gynecol Reprod Biol 2004; 114:92–6.

29. Radpour CJ, Keenan JA. Consecutive cervical pregnancies. Fertil Steril 2004; 81:210–13.

12

Managing non-tubal ectopic pregnancy: interstitial and cervical pregnancy

Emma Kirk

Introduction • Interstitial pregnancies • Cervical pregnancies • Practical points

INTRODUCTION

We have heard already in detail about the management options for tubal ectopic pregnancies. However although non-tubal ectopic pregnancies account for only 5% of all ectopic pregnancies, they contribute to a disproportionate number of serious complications.[1] Both diagnosis and management can pose a significant problem. In the past many were not diagnosed until the time of surgery, which was often associated with serious morbidity and mortality. The most commonly encountered non-tubal ectopic pregnancies are interstitial and cervical pregnancies. Although rare, other types of non-tubal ectopic pregnancies include ovarian, abdominal and caesarean section scar pregnancies.

INTERSTITIAL PREGNANCIES

Interstitial pregnancies have been reported to account for between 1 and 6% of all ectopic pregnancies.[2,3] An interstitial pregnancy occurs when the pregnancy implants outside of the endometrial cavity, within the interstitial part of the myometrium. It has been reported that in 20% of cases that progress beyond 12 weeks' gestation, life-threatening rupture of the uterus can occur with a mortality rate of 2.5%.[4] In the *Why Mothers Die* report 2000–2002, four out of the 11 deaths from ruptured ectopic pregnancies were due to interstitial pregnancies.[5]

Aetiological factors are similar to those for tubal ectopic pregnancies; however, women with a history of previous salpingectomy are at increased risk. In 32 cases reported to the Canadian registry of the Society of Reproductive surgeons, 37.5% of patients had a history of ipsilateral salpingectomy.[6]

Diagnosis

Historically interstitial pregnancies were usually diagnosed intraoperatively; however, using transvaginal ultrasonography (TVS) the diagnosis is now most commonly made before the time of rupture. The following ultrasonographic criteria are used: (1) a regular endometrial echo, with no visible gestational sac within it; (2) products of conception located outside of the endometrial echo and surrounded by a continuous rim of myometrium, within the interstitial area (Figure 12.1).[7]

Management

As is touched on in Chapter 11, surgical management is an important option and in the past has always been the mainstay of treatment. Due to the location of the pregnancy, laparotomy with

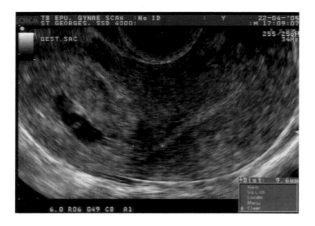

Figure 12.1 A transvaginal ultrasound image of a right interstitial pregnancy and an empty uterine cavity. (Reproduced from G. Condous, E. Okaro, T. Bourne. The conservative management of early pregnancy complications: a review of the literature. Ultrasound Obstet Gynecol 2003; 22:420–430, with permission from John Wiley and Sons Ltd.)

Table 12.1. Summary of success of methotrexate in the management of interstitial pregnancies – a review of the literature

Year	Author	Number of cases	Route of methotrexate administration	Initial hCG (range) (IU/L)	Success rate – successful resolution without surgery	Overall success	Comments
1991	Fernandez[11]	4	Systemic – multiple dose		75% (3/4)	67%	1 case also received systemic methotrexate
		2	Local		50% (1/2)		
1992	Karsdorp[12]	5	Systemic – multiple dose	1500–16 800	100%(5/5)	100%	1 patient received 2 doses, 3 patients required 3 doses. 1 required local methotrexate
1996	Benifla[13]	6	Systemic – multiple dose	364–43 000	66% (4/6)	83%	1 case received a local dose of methotrexate
		6	Local	360–10 000	100% (6/6)		
1996	Hajenius[14]	8	Systemic – multiple dose	410–81 000	100% (8/8)	100%	3 required a second dose
1997	Timor-Tritsch[15]	7	Local		100% (7/7)	100%	1 case needed a laparoscopy for haemostasis
1999	Hafner[16]	5	Systemic – multiple dose	793–41 150	80% (4/5)	90%	
		5	Local	102–16 400	100% (5/5)		
2004	Jermy[7]	17	Systemic – single dose	32–31 381	94% (16/17)	94%	6 cases required a second dose
2005	Dilbaz[17]	3	Systemic – single dose		100% (3/3)	100%	
2005	Monteagudo[18]	2	Local	11 000–62 000	100% (2/2)	67%	1 also had systemic methotrexate
		1	Systemic – single dose	29 200	0% (0/1)		Also received local injection of KCl

cornual resection or hysterectomy is often the outcome. Cornual resection has marked effects on future fertility as it leads to an increased risk of uterine rupture in future pregnancies. Less-invasive surgical options including laparoscopic cornual resection, tubal curettage and combined hysteroscopic and laparoscopic resection have been reported.[8–10]

Today most unruptured interstitial pregnancies should be managed non-surgically. Methotrexate has been shown to be safe and effective in managing unruptured interstitial pregnancies. Table 12.1 summarizes some of the published literature on the use of methotrexate in such pregnancies. As for tubal ectopic pregnancies, methotrexate can be given systemically, using either a single-dose or multiple-dose regimen, or locally under transvaginal ultrasound guidance or at the time of laparoscopy (see Chapter 11). Overall success rates vary from 67 to 100%.[7,11–18] Interstitial pregnancies can also be treated by local injection of potassium chloride. This is particularly useful in more advanced ectopic pregnancies, in viable pregnancies or heterotopic pregnancies.[18]

Suggested management protocol

If a woman diagnosed with an interstitial pregnancy is haemodynamically unstable or in pain, surgery should be the primary treatment. Anecdotally these ectopic pregnancies tend to rupture at a later stage and with greater immediate blood loss. A large-bore intravenous cannula should be inserted and blood sent for full blood count, serum hCG and group and save. Ideally 4 units of blood should be cross-matched. Surgery should ideally be laparoscopic and as conservative as possible in the form of a cornuostomy or cornual resection. However, laparotomy is more likely than with tubal ectopic pregnancies, reflecting the degree of blood loss that may be encountered and the degree of surgical difficulty. In asymptomatic, haemodynamically stable women, management should be non-surgical. As previously described, a bimanual examination should be performed to exclude cervical excitation and adnexal tenderness. Blood should be sent for full blood count, serum hCG and progesterone, liver and renal function tests

and group and save. If there is no fetal cardiac activity on TVS, single-dose systemic methotrexate (50 mg/m^2) is the treatment of choice. This should be administered and followed up according to the protocol used for tubal ectopic pregnancies that is described in detail in Chapter 10. This form of treatment can be managed on an outpatient basis with the same warnings given to the patient. If there is fetal cardiac activity or the gestation is advanced, management should be with local injection of methotrexate or potassium chloride under TVS guidance. This can be carried out under general anaesthetic as a day case, however, observation in hospital may be wise until there is no fetal cardiac activity. TVS examinations should be repeated every 2 days until the cessation of fetal cardiac activity. Follow up should be with repeat serum hCG estimations as for systemic methotrexate. Multiple-dose systemic methotrexate, as also described in Chapter 10, is an option if there is no operator available to administer it locally (Figure 12.2).

CASE REPORT

A 34-year-old woman attended the Early Pregnancy Unit (EPU) with a history of lower abdominal pain and light vaginal spotting. Her one previous pregnancy resulted in a spontaneous vaginal delivery at term. She was 6^{+3} weeks' gestation according to her last menstrual period. This was an unplanned pregnancy. She had had a transabdominal ultrasound scan performed at a termination clinic 2 days previously, which did not show any evidence of an intrauterine pregnancy. A TVS performed in the EPU showed an empty uterine cavity with a gestational sac measuring 29 × 23 mm in the left cornual region (Figure 12.3). A diagnosis of a left interstitial ectopic pregnancy was made and blood was taken to measure serum human chorionic gonadotrophin (hCG) and progesterone. The serum hCG was 2660 IU/L and progesterone 4 nmol/L. A single injection of methotrexate was given at a dose of 50 mg/m^2. On days 4 and 7 following methotrexate the hCG levels were 2197 IU/L and 1839 IU/L respectively. As the hCG had decreased by 16% between days 4 and 7, the hCG level was

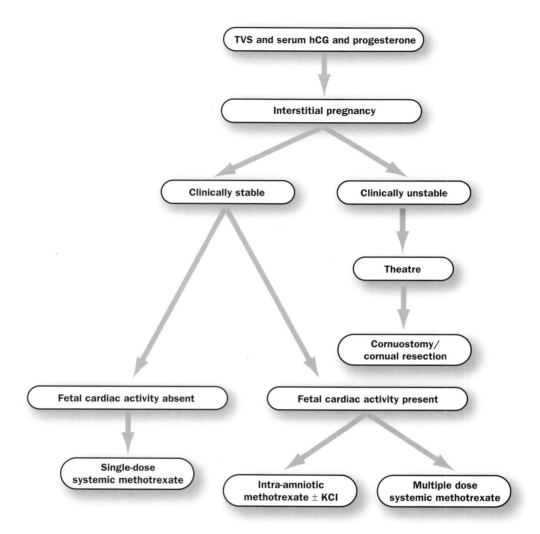

Figure 12.2 Flow diagram to illustrate a suggested management plan for interstitial pregnancies.

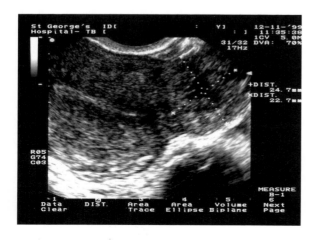

Figure 12.3 A transvaginal ultrasound image showing a left interstitial pregnancy. (Reproduced from G. Condous, E. Okaro, T. Bourne. The conservative management of early pregnancy complications: a review of the literature. Ultrasound Obstet Gynecol 2003; 22:420–430, with permission from John Wiley and Sons Ltd.)

repeated in 1 week. The hCG level was then checked on a weekly basis. She had a successful resolution of her ectopic pregnancy as defined by an hCG of <10 IU/L within 7 weeks of her presentation to the EPU. A TVS repeated 3 months after treatment showed only a minimal residual mass in the left uterine cornu.

CERVICAL PREGNANCIES

Cervical pregnancies account for less than 1% of all ectopic pregnancies with a reported incidence of between 1 in 10 000 to 1 in 95 000 pregnancies.[19] It occurs when the pregnancy implants into the cervical mucosa, below the level of the internal os. Historically women with a cervical ectopic pregnancy underwent hysterectomy and it was only at the time of pathological examination of the uterus that a diagnosis was confirmed.

The exact aetiology of cervical pregnancy is unknown. One suggested theory is that there is rapid transport of the fertilized ovum to the cervical canal before it is capable of nidation.[20] Trauma to the cervix and endometrial lining during operative uterine procedures has also been implicated.[20] Previous surgical termination of pregnancy and Asherman's syndrome are recognized risk factors.[21,22] Like tubal ectopic pregnancies, cervical pregnancies are also associated with assisted reproductive techniques.

Diagnosis

In 1911, Rubin proposed pathological criteria for the diagnosis of cervical ectopic pregnancy after hysterectomy: (1) cervical glands must be present opposite the placental attachment, (2) the attachment of the placenta to the cervix must be intimate; (3) the whole or a portion of the placenta must be situated below the entrance of the uterine vessels, or below the peritoneal reflection of the anterior and posterior surface of the uterus; and (4) no fetal elements are present in the corpus uteri.[23] The first report of a cervical ectopic pregnancy diagnosed using ultrasound was in 1978.[24] Since then ultrasonographic criteria, not too dissimilar to Rubin's original criteria, have been developed to diagnose cervical pregnancy. The

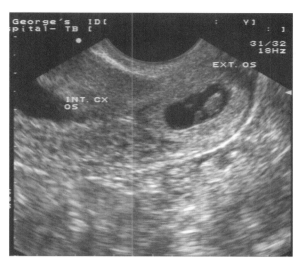

Figure 12.4 A transvaginal scan image showing a cervical ectopic pregnancy. (Reproduced from G. Condous, E. Okaro, T. Bourne. The conservative management of early pregnancy complications: a review of the literature. Ultrasound Obstet Gynecol 2003; 22:420–430, with permission from John Wiley and Sons Ltd.)

criteria aim to distinguish between an early intrauterine pregnancy, an ongoing miscarriage with a gestational sac passing through the cervix and a cervical ectopic pregnancy. At present the following criteria using transvaginal ultrasonography are: (1) an empty uterus; (2) a barrel-shaped cervix; (3) a gestational sac present below the level of the uterine arteries; (4) the absence of the 'sliding sign' (when pressure is applied to the cervix using the probe in a miscarriage, the gestational sac slides against the endocervical canal but does not in an implanted cervical pregnancy); and (5) blood flow around the gestation sac using colour Doppler (Figure 12.4).[25,26]

Management

Traditionally cervical pregnancies have been managed surgically – an approach that is notoriously hazardous. As a consequence, many women with this type of ectopic pregnancy underwent hysterectomy. As cervical pregnancies can now be detected earlier in asymptomatic women conservative treatment is an option. A conservative surgical approach

Table 12.2. Summary and success of conservative management of cervical pregnancies – a review of the literature. (Reproduced from [54] © Intrnational Society of Ultrasound in Obstetrics and Gynecology, first published by John Wiley & Sons Ltd.)

Case	Author	Year	N =	Gestation (days)	CRL (mm)	FH	Local treatment	Systemic MTX	Curettage	Successful conservative management	Other comments
1	Mitra[33]	2000	1	76		+	MTX, KCl	Yes		Yes	
2	Pascual[34]	2001	1			+		Yes	Yes	Yes	Twin cervical pregnancy
3	Goldberg[35]	2000	1			+		Yes		Yes	
4	Margolis[36]	2000	1	42				Yes	Yes	Yes	
5	Has[37]	2001	1	74			MTX	Yes	Yes	Yes	Additional systemic dose and bilateral uterine artery embolisation
6	Melili[38]	2001	1	56				Yes		Yes	Twin cervical and cervico-isthmic pregnancy
7	Tuncer[39]	2001	1	72					Yes	No	Uterine artery ligation, cervical hysterotomy then TAH performed due to uncontrolled bleeding
8	Mashiach[31]	2002	4	44				Yes		Yes	Emergency insertion of Shirodkar cerclage
9				44				Yes		Yes	Emergency insertion of Shirodkar cerclage
10				45						Yes	Primary treatment – elective insertion of Shirodkar cerclage
11				59						Yes	Primary treatment – elective insertion of Shirodkar cerclage
12	Chew[40]	2001	2	61	19	+		Yes		Yes	Prostaglandin (sulprostone) given with the MTX
13				49	6	+		Yes		Yes	Prostaglandin (sulprostone) given with the MTX
14	Gun[41]	2002	1	49	9.1	+		Yes		Yes	Bilateral uterine artery embolization
15	Jeong[42]	2003	1	35		+	MTX	Yes		Yes	Triplet cervical pregnacy, one viable fetus
16	Celik[19]	2003	1	42			MTX	Yes		Yes	
17	Lin[43]	2003	3	42			MTX			Yes	Laparoscopic bilateral uterine artery ligation
18				49			MTX			Yes	Laparoscopic bilateral uterine artery ligation
19				63			MTX			Yes	Laparoscopic bilateral uterine artery ligation
20	Leon[44]	2003	1	49	9.9	+		Yes	Yes	Yes	Foley catheter balloon tamponade
21	Suzumori[45]	2003	1	77				Yes		Yes	Cervical cerclage, uterine artery ligation, unilateral internal iliac artery ligation
22	Sherer[46]	2003	1			+		Yes		Yes	Uterine artery embolization
23	Gianetto-Berruti[47]	2004	1	42				Yes		Yes	
24	Cepni[48]	2004	1					Yes	Yes	Yes	
25	Hidalgo[49]	2004	1	63				Yes	Yes	Yes	Methotrexate after curettage
26	Sherer[50]	2004	1	81				Yes		Yes	
27	Yazici[51]	2004	1	49		+	KCl, MTX			Yes	
28	Kim[52]	2004	31	6		–			Yes	Yes	
29				91		–			Yes	No	TAH due to prolonged bleeding
30				84		–			Yes	Yes	Vasopressin
31				43		–			Yes	Yes	Re-curettage due to prolonged bleeding

#	Author	Year	n	Meas1	Meas2	Sign	Drug			Outcome	Notes
32				42		−			Yes	No	TAH – due to prolonged bleeding
33				49		−			Yes	No	TAH – due to rupture of lower uterine segment
34				52		+			Yes	Yes	Ligation of uterine arteries
35				47		+			Yes	Yes	Foley catheter balloon tamponade
36				48		+			Yes	Yes	
37				41		+		Yes	Yes	Yes	Laparotomy
38				41		+		Yes		Yes	
39				48		+		Yes		Yes	
40				42		+		Yes	Yes	Yes	
41				42		+		Yes	Yes	Yes	
42				48		+		Yes		Yes	
43				42		+		Yes	Yes	Yes	
44				49		+	MTX	Yes		Yes	
45				49		+	MTX	Yes		Yes	
46				69		+	MTX	Yes	Yes	Yes	Hypogastric artery ligation, Foley catheter balloon tamponade
47				59		+		Yes	Yes	Yes	
48				38		−		Yes		Yes	
49				40		−		Yes		Yes	
50				49		−		Yes		Yes	
51				42		−		Yes		Yes	
52				41		−		Yes		Yes	
53				35		−		Yes		Yes	
54				40		−		Yes		Yes	
55				54		−		Yes		Yes	
56				40		−		Yes		Yes	
57				43		−		Yes	Yes	Yes	
58				35		−		Yes	Yes	Yes	Cervical cerclage, ligation of uterine arteries
59	Monteagudo[18]	2005	10	52	11	+	MTX	Yes		Yes	Required a second dose
60				73	36	+	KCl	Yes		Yes	
61				41	3.3	+	KCl	Yes		Yes	
62				44	6.7	+	KCl	Yes		Yes	
63				42	4	+	KCl	Yes		Yes	
64				71	23.2	+	KCl	Yes		Yes	
65				43	5	+	MTX			Yes	
66				49	9.4	+	KCl	Yes	Yes	Yes	Thrombocytopenia
67				42	4	+	KCl			Yes	Heterotopic
68				49	10	+	KCl			Yes	Heterotopic
69	Hassiakos[53]	2005	6	35+		−	MTX		Yes	Yes	Curettage performed as a definitive treatment
70				35+		−	MTX		Yes	Yes	Curettage performed as a definitive treatment
71				35+		−	MTX		Yes	Yes	Curettage performed as a definitive treatment
72				35+		−	MTX		Yes	Yes	Curettage performed as a definitive treatment
73				42+		+	MTX		Yes	Yes	Curettage performed as a definitive treatment
74				56+		+	MTX		Yes	Yes	Curettage performed as a definitive treatment

such as dilatation and curettage has been reported to be successful in some cases.[27] However, because of the risk of haemorrhage, techniques are needed to reduce bleeding after curettage. Reported methods include: uterine artery embolization,[27] uterine artery ligation and cervicotomy,[28] Foley catheter tamponade,[29] local prostaglandin injection[30] and the use of cervical sutures.[31] More important has been the shift towards the use of non-surgical management. As with interstitial pregnancies, methotrexate has revolutionized the management of cervical pregnancies. Again it can be given systemically using either a single- or multiple-dose regimen, or locally under ultrasound guidance. The choice of regimen will depend on the serum hCG level, the size of the ectopic mass and the presence or absence of fetal cardiac activity. A review of 52 cases managed with either systemic or local methotrexate had an overall success rate of 61.5% for primary methotrexate treatment.[32] Fetal cardiac activity has been shown to be associated with a higher rate of primary methotrexate failure. So too has an initial serum hCG level of greater than 10 000 IU/L, a gestational age of more than 9 weeks and a crown–rump length of greater than 10 mm.[32]

Table 12.2 summarizes 24 studies and case reports published since 2000 on the management of cervical pregnancies.[18,19,33–54] It can be seen that there are a variety of accepted methods of managing them. The overall success of conservative management in the 74 individual cases is 94.6% (70/74) with only 5.4% (4/74) of women needing a hysterectomy. However 20.3% (15/74) of women needed an additional procedure to control bleeding, such as uterine artery embolization, Foley catheter balloon tamponade or the insertion of a Shirodkar suture.

Suggested management protocol

How a cervical pregnancy should be managed will depend on the gestation, clinical signs and symptoms and the presence or absence of fetal cardiac activity (Figure 12.5). For non-viable pregnancies it is appropriate to give a single intramuscular injection of methotrexate at a dose of 50 mg/m^2, as detailed above and in Chapter 10. For cervical pregnancies with fetal cardiac activity, the first-line management should ideally be intra-amniotic potassium chloride or methotrexate given under ultrasound guidance, as above. This procedure involves a certain level of expertise, and if that is not available multiple-dose systemic treatment may be an appropriate alternative. Surgical intervention should be reserved for those with failed medical management or those who are bleeding heavily. It should be in the form of dilatation and curettage ideally under ultrasound guidance. If the procedure is complicated by uncontrolled bleeding, insertion of a cervical suture or a Foley catheter balloon tamponade can be effective. In any unit managing cervical pregnancies close liaison with an interventional radiologist is important in case of the need for procedures such as uterine artery embolization.

CASE REPORT

A 38-year-old primiparous woman presented to the Early Pregnancy Unit with a 2-day history of painless light vaginal bleeding. She had a positive pregnancy test and was 6^{+0} weeks' gestation according to her last menstrual period. It was her second pregnancy. Her first pregnancy was terminated surgically at 7 weeks' gestation. A transvaginal scan (TVS) performed on the day of presentation revealed a gestational sac implanted in the cervix below the level of the uterine arteries. It contained a viable fetal pole measuring 3 mm. The serum hCG level was 6249 IU/L. A decision was made to give intra-amniotic methotrexate. A 16-gauge double-lumen oocyte collection needle (Casmed, Banstead, Surrey, England) was introduced under TVS guidance into the amniotic sac. Amniotic fluid was withdrawn initially and followed by administration of 25 mg methotrexate into the amniotic sac. She was kept as an inpatient overnight and rescanned the next day. On repeat TVS no fetal cardiac activity was seen and the sac had been disrupted. She was discharged home that day. She was followed up for a total of 74 days, by which time her serum hCG level was <10 IU/L. Heavy bleeding did not complicate her management and she did not have any side effects from the methotrexate.

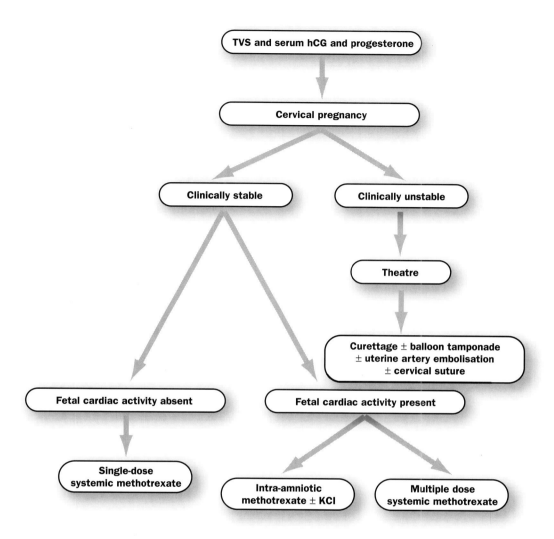

Figure 12.5 Flow diagram to illustrate a suggested management plan for cervical pregnancies.

PRACTICAL POINTS

1. Although only 5% of all ectopic pregnancies are non-tubal, they are responsible for a disproportionate amount of morbidity and mortality.
2. Surgery is hazardous due to the anatomical location of the pregnancies and often results in hysterectomy.
3. The aim should be to manage the majority non-surgically.
4. Single dose systemic methotrexate should be the treatment of choice for non-viable non-tubal ectopic pregnancies.
5. Local injection of methotrexate or potassium chloride is the treatment of choice for viable or more advanced ectopic gestations.

REFERENCES

1. Condous G. The management of early pregnancy complications. Best Pract Res Clin Obstet Gynaecol 2004; 18:37–57.

2. Rock JA, Thompson JD, eds. Telinde's Operative Gynecology, 8th edn. Philadelphia: Lippincott-Raven, 1997:505–20.

3. Fernandez H, De Zeigler D, Bourget P, Feltain P, Frydman R. The place of methotrexate in the management of interstitial pregnancy. Hum Reprod 1991; 6:1271–9.

4. Kucera E, Helbich TH, Klem I, et al. Systemic methotrexate treatment of interstitial pregnancy – magnetic resonance imaging (MRI) as a valuable tool for monitoring treatment. Wien Klin Wochenschr 2000; 112(17):772–5.

5. 'Why Mothers Die', Triennial Report 2000–2002. Confidential Enquiry into Maternal Deaths, UK.

6. Tulandi T, Al-Jaroudi D. Interstitial pregnancy: results from the Society of Reproductive Surgeons Registry. Obstet Gynecol 2004; 103:47–50.

7. Jermy K, Thomas J, Doo A, Bourne T. The conservative management of interstitial pregnancy. Br J Obstet Gynaecol 2004; 111:1283–8.

8. Chan LY, Yuen PM. Successful treatment of ruptured interstitial pregnancy with laparoscopic surgery. A report of 2 cases. J Reprod Med 2003; 48:569–71.

9. Ayoubi J, Fanchin R, Olivennes F, Fernandez H, Pons J. Tubal curettage: a new conservative treatment for haemorrhagic interstitial pregnancies. Hum Reprod 2001; 16:780–1.

10. Katz D, Barrett J, Sanfilippo J, Badway D. Combined hysteroscopy and laparoscopy in the treatment of interstitial pregnancy. Am J Obstet Gynecol 2003; 188:1113–4.

11. Fernandez H, De Zeigler D, Bourget P, Feltain P, Frydman R. The place of methotrexate in the management of interstitial pregnancy. Hum Reprod 1991; 6:302–6.

12. Karsdorp VH, Van der Veen F, Schats R, Boer-Meisel ME, Kenemans P. Successful treatment with methotrexate of five interstitial pregnancies. Hum Reprod 1992; 7:1164–9.

13. Benifla JL, Fernandez H, Sebban E, et al. Alternative to surgery of treatment of unruptured interstitial pregnancies: 15 cases of medical management. Eur J Obstet Gynaecol Reprod Biol 1996; 70:151–6.

14. Hajenius PJ, Voight RR, Engelsbel S, et al. Serum human chorionic gonadotrophin clearance curves in patients with interstitial pregnancy treated with systemic methotrexate. Fertil Steril 1996; 66:723–8.

15. Timor-Tritsch IE, Monteagudo A, Lerner JP. A 'potentially safer' route for puncture and injection of cornual ectopic pregnancies. Ultrasound Obstet Gynaecol 1997; 7:353–5.

16. Hafner T, Aslam N, Ross JA, Zosmer N, Jurkovic D. The effectiveness of non-surgical management of early interstitial pregnancy: a report of ten cases and review of the literature. Ultrasound Obstet Gynaecol 1999; 13:131–6.

17. Dilbaz S, Katas B, Demir B, Dilbaz B. Treating cornual pregnancy with a single methotrexate injection: a report of 3 cases. J Reprod Med 2005; 50:141–4.

18. Monteagudo A, Minior VK, Stephenson C, Monda S, Timor-Tritsch IE. Non-surgical management of live ectopic pregnancy with ultrasound-guided local injection: a case series. Ultrasound Obstet Gynaecol 2005; 25:282–8.

19. Celik C, Bala A, Acar A, Gezgine K, Akyurek C. Methotrexate for cervical pregnancy. A case report. J Reprod Med 2003; 48:130–2.

20. Studdiford WE. Cervical pregnancy: a partial review of the literature and a report of two probable cases. Am J Obstet Gynaecol 1945; 49:169.

21. Shinagawa S, Nagayama M. Cervical pregnancy as a possible sequela of induced abortion. Report of 19 cases. Am J Obstet Gynaecol 1969; 105(2):282–4.

22. Dicker D, Feldberg D, Samuel N, Goldman JA. Etiology of cervical pregnancy. Association with abortion, pelvic pathology, IUDs and Asherman's syndrome. J Reprod Med 1985; 30(1):25–7.

23. Rubin IC. Cervical pregnancy. Surg Gynecol Obstet 1911; 13:625.

24. Raskin MM. Diagnosis of cervical pregnancy by ultrasound. A case report. Am J Obstet Gynaecol 1978; 130:234

25. Jurkovic D, Hackett E, Campbell S. Diagnosis and treatment of early cervical pregnancy: a review and a report of two cases treated conservatively. Ultrasound Obstet Gynaecol 1996; 8:373–80.

26. Timor-Tritsch IE, Monteagudo A, Mandeville EO, et al. Successful management of viable cervical pregnancy by local injection of methotrexate guided by transvaginal ultrasonography. Am J Obstet Gynecol 1994; 170:737–9.

27. Frates MC, Benson CB, Doubilet PM, et al. Cervical ectopic pregnancy: results of conservative treatment. Radiology 1994; 191(3):773–5.

28. Su TH, Wang YD, Chen CP, Lei SY. A conservative surgical treatment of cervical pregnancy with active bleeding – uterine artery ligation and cervicotomy. Int J Gynaecol Obstet 1992; 4:275–9.

29. Fylstra DL, Coffey MD. Treatment of cervical pregnancy with cerclage, curettage and balloon tamponade. A report of three cases. J Reprod Med 2001; 46:71–4.

30. Spitzer D, Steiner H, Graf A, Zajc M, Staudach A. Conservative treatment of cervical pregnancy by curet-

tage and local prostaglandin injection. Hum Reprod 1997; 12:860–6.

31. Mashiach S, Admon D, Oelsner G, et al. Cervical Shirodkar cerclage may be the treatment modality of choice for cervical pregnancy. Hum Reprod 2002; 17:493–6.

32. Hung TH, Shau WY, Hsieh TT, et al. Prognostic factors for an unsatisfactory primary methotrexate treatment of cervical pregnancy: a quantitative review. Hum Reprod 1998; 12:2636–42.

33. Mitra AG, Harris-Owens M. Conservative medical management of advanced cervical ectopic pregnancies. Obstet Gynecol Surv 2000; 55:385–9.

34. Pascual MA, Ruiz J, Tresserra F, et al. Cervical ectopic twin pregnancy: diagnosis and conservative treatment: case report. Hum Reprod 2001; 16:584–6.

35. Goldberg JM, Widrich T. Successful management of a viable cervical pregnancy by single-dose methotrexate. J Womens Health Gend Based Med 2000; 9:43–5.

36. Margolis K. Cervical pregnancy treated with a single intravenous administration of methotrexate plus oral folinic acid. Aust NZ J Obstet Gynaecol 2000; 40:347–9.

37. Has R, Balci NC, Ibrahimoglu L, Rozanes I, Topuz S. Uterine artery embolization in a 10–week cervical pregnancy with coexisting fibroids. Int J Gynaecol Obstet 2001; 72:253–8.

38. Melilli GA, Cormio G, Putignano G, Loverro G, Selvaggi L. Successful treatment of cervical and simultaneous cervico-isthmic pregnancy with methotrexate. Clin Exp Obstet Gynecol 2001; 28:89–90.

39. Tuncer R, Uygur D, Kis S, et al. Inevitable hysterectomy despite conservative surgical management in advanced cervical pregnancy: a case report. Eur J Obstet Gynecol Reprod Biol 2001; 100:102–4.

40. Chew S, Anandakumar C. Medical management of cervical pregnancy – a report of two cases. Singapore Med J 2001; 42:537–9.

41. Gun M, Mavrogiorgis M. Cervical ectopic pregnancy: a case report and literature review. Ultrasound Obstet Gynecol 2002; 19:297–301.

42. Jeong EH, Kim YB, Ji IW, Kim HS. Triplet cervical pregnancy treated with intraamniotic methotrexate. Obstet Gynecol 2002; 100:1117–9.

43. Lin H, Kung FT. Combination of laparoscopic bilateral uterine artery ligation and intraamniotic methotrexate injection for conservative management of cervical pregnancy. J Am Assoc Gynecol Laparosc 2003; 10:215–8.

44. Leon G, Hidalgo L, Chedraui P. Cervical pregnancy: transvaginal sonographic diagnosis and conservative surgical management after failure of systemic methotrexate. Ultrasound Obstet Gynecol 2003; 21:620–2.

45. Suzumori N, Katano K, Sato T, et al. Conservative treatment by angiographic artery embolization of an 11-week cervical pregnancy after a period of heavy bleeding. Fertil Steril 2003; 80:617–19.

46. Sherer DM, Lysikiewicz A, Abulafia O. Viable cervical pregnancy managed with systemic methotrexate, uterine artery embolization, and local tamponade with inflated Foley catheter balloon. Am J Perinatol 2003; 20:263–7.

47. Gianetto-Berruti A, Feyles V, Mohide PT. Medical management of a cervical pregnancy: a case report. J Obstet Gynaecol Can 2003; 25:858–60.

48. Cepni I, Ocal P, Erkan S, Erzik B. Conservative treatment of cervical ectopic pregnancy with transvaginal ultrasound-guided aspiration and single-dose methotrexate. Fertil Steril 2004; 81:1130–2.

49. Hidalgo LA, Penafiel J, Chedraui PA. Management of cervical pregnancy: risk factors for failed systemic methotrexate. J Perinat Med 2004; 32:184–6.

50. Sherer DM, Dalloul M, Santoso P, et al. Complete abortion of a nonviable cervical pregnancy following methotrexate treatment. Am J Perinatol 2004; 21:223–6.

51. Yazici G, Aban M, Arslan M, Pata O, Oz U. Treatment of a cervical viable pregnancy with a single intraamniotic methotrexate injection: a case report. Arch Gynecol Obstet 2004; 270:61–3.

52. Kim TJ, Seong SJ, Lee KJ, et al. Clinical outcomes of patients treated for cervical pregnancy with or without methotrexate. J Korean Med Sci 2004; 19:848–52.

53. Hassiakos D, Bakas P, Creatsas G. Cervical pregnancy treated with transvaginal ultrasound-guided intraamniotic instillation of methotrexate. Arch Gynecol Obstet 2005; 271:69–72.

54. Kirk E, Condous G, Haider Z, et al. The conservative management of cervical ectopic pregnancies. Ultrasound Obstet Gynecol 2006; 27:430–7.

13

Caesarean scar pregnancy

Cecilia Bottomley

Introduction • Incidence • Risk factors • Symptoms and signs • Diagnosis and investigations • Natural history of Caesarean scar pregnancy • Management • Future pregnancies • A proposed management strategy • Case report • Practical points

INTRODUCTION

A caesarean scar pregnancy is a pregnancy within the myometrial scar of a previous caesarean section. It is an iatrogenic entity, whereby the blastocyst enters a microscopic tract in the uterine scar and implants in the deficient anterior uterine wall. The pathogenesis is similar to other cases of intramural ectopic pregnancy that may occur after uterine surgery such as manual removal of placenta, uterine curettage or myomectomy.[1]

Caesarean scar pregnancy was first described in 1978 by Larsen, where a case was treated with laparotomy, hysterotomy resection and scar dehiscence repair.[2] However most reports have been published since 1995. This perhaps reflects the increase in the routine use of transvaginal ultrasound for suspected early pregnancy pathology and the increase in caesarean section rates to above 20% in many countries over the last few decades.

INCIDENCE

Caesarean scar pregnancy is considered to be the rarest form of ectopic pregnancy. However the incidence is reported to be as high as 1 in 1800 to 1 in 2216 in some studies.[3,4] Seow reports scar pregnancies comprising 6.1% of all ectopic pregnancies in women with a previous caesarean section (overall caesarean rate in their tertiary

centre being 30%) and a rate of caesarean scar pregnancy of 0.15% of all pregnant women who have had a previous caesarean section. However these studies may be open to selection bias, and the real incidence in the general 'post-section' population is not known.

RISK FACTORS

Multiple previous caesarean sections are associated with a higher risk for a caesarean scar pregnancy. Previous dilatation and curettage, placenta praevia, ectopic pregnancy and in vitro fertilization are other reported associations.[5,6]

Previous caesarean section for breech presentation is more common than might be expected and it is postulated that this may be because the lower segment of the uterus does not develop fully in a breech presentation, thus predisposing to suboptimal healing of the uterine incision after caesarean section and a greater exposed surface area of myometrium for implantation of a scar pregnancy.

One case of caesarean scar pregnancy has been reported after the failure of the progesterone only emergency contraceptive.[7]

SYMPTOMS AND SIGNS

Most women present with vaginal bleeding varying from light spotting to life-threatening haemorrhage.[3] Some women also report lower abdominal pain. The women may also be asymptomatic with the condition recognized at the time of a routine scan in the first trimester.

Initial misdiagnosis of a scar ectopic pregnancy as intrauterine is common. Thus women may undergo attempted evacuation of retained products of conception (for presumed miscarriage) or suction termination of pregnancy (for presumed intrauterine pregnancy) where the diagnosis of caesarean scar pregnancy has not been suspected. Profuse haemorrhage can result, often as the sac is disrupted by the curettage. These women present as emergencies and need immediate surgical intervention.

Most women, however, are haemodynamically stable at presentation. Speculum examination may show blood in the vagina. The cervix usually appears normal, though bimanual examination may reveal an anterior uterine swelling (possibly displaced to the right or left), with or without tenderness.

DIAGNOSIS AND INVESTIGATIONS

The diagnosis of caesarean scar pregnancy is made by transvaginal ultrasonography. The absence of an intrauterine pregnancy and an empty cervical canal are accompanied by the presence of a gestational sac implanted within the lower anterior segment of uterine corpus, with evidence of myometrial dehiscence. If the depth of invasion into the myometrial scar is small, there may be some continuation between the sac and the uterine cavity. Alternatively, if the sac is deeply embedded in the scar, the sac may be seen bulging towards the urinary bladder, with only a very thin myometrial layer visible between the sac and the bladder. Diagnosis may be difficult in the presence of uterine fibroids that can obscure the view.

Prominent peritrophoblastic flow may be shown with Doppler ultrasound featuring high velocity and low impedance. Caesarean scar pregnancies have also been described with three-dimensional ultrasound imaging, though the advantages of this method over conventional B-mode scanning have not been proven.[8] Similarly, magnetic resonance imaging and transabdominal ultrasound scans have been used to aid assessment, particularly with respect to assessing the integrity of the myometrium between the pregnancy sac and the bladder. However in most women such modalities are not necessary for an accurate diagnosis to be made.

Caesarean scar pregnancies tend to be diagnosed between 5 and 12 weeks.[3] Beyond this gestation, a pregnancy is likely to appear to be intrauterine if the depth of invasion of the myometrium is small, or to be an abdominal pregnancy if it extrudes very anteriorly through the myometrium.

The differential diagnosis for a caesarean scar pregnancy includes a cervical pregnancy or a miscarriage, with the sac in the lower uterus or cervix. As discussed in Chapter 12, with a cervical pregnancy, the cervix appears dilated ('ballooning'), with the sac visualized within it. In the case of a miscarriage, the sac is usually distorted or collapsed and the 'sliding sign' may be present (apparent sliding of the sac up and down the cervix or uterine cavity with pressure from the transvaginal probe).

Serum human chorionic gonadotrophin (hCG) and progesterone should be taken when the diagnosis of caesarean scar pregnancy is suspected, as a baseline by which to monitor the regression of the pregnancy with treatment, rather than as a diagnostic aid. Serum for group and save should be taken due to the risk of significant haemorrhage and renal and liver function should be checked if methotrexate therapy is to be considered.

NATURAL HISTORY OF CAESAREAN SCAR PREGNANCY

The natural history of caesarean scar pregnancy is not fully known. Unlike a cervical pregnancy, a caesarean scar pregnancy may potentially be carried to term, though this is likely to be associated with significant morbidity and possibly mortality. The known association between multiple caesarean sections and an increased risk of abnormally implanted placentae (praevia, accreta and percreta) suggests that if a caesarean scar pregnancy were to continue to term, then it would be associated with such placental pathology. Indeed many cases of abnormal placentation reported in the past may well have been unrecognized caesarean scar pregnancies. It therefore seems likely that this is not a new condition, but the earlier recognition of an old problem. Life-threatening haemorrhage, coagulopathy and hysterectomy at or after delivery are significant risks for such women.

There have however been several case reports where women have been managed expectantly. Ben Nagi recently reported a case of first-trimester diagnosis of caesarean scar pregnancy that was managed expectantly to term (due to patient reluctance to undergo earlier termination) with the development of placenta praevia and accreta.[9] Maymon describes another case that proceeded to 35 weeks when emergency caesarean hysterectomy was performed.[5]

Earlier complications may also occur. Jurkovic's three reported cases of expectant management of caesarean scar pregnancy all resulted in spontaneous fetal loss.[4] The first loss occurred at 10 weeks with an incomplete miscarriage, the second at 10 weeks, subsequently treated with systemic methotrexate and the third resulting in miscarriage at 17 weeks with severe bleeding necessitating hysterectomy.

Liang reports a case of uterine rupture in the first trimester due to a caesarean scar pregnancy.[10] Marcus reports a similar case where a woman presented with abdominal pain and bleeding at 13 weeks' gestation.[11] In this case an ultrasound scan suggested dehiscence of the previous caesarean section scar with a viable pregnancy within the scar tissue between the uterus and bladder. Subsequent hysterectomy, after embolization of the uterine arteries, confirmed complete rupture of the lower uterine segment and placenta percreta.

It may be, as discussed by Maymon, that there is a distinction between those scar pregnancies shallowly embedded within the scar with protrusion of the sac towards the uterine cavity which may be viable to the third trimester, though this still presents the risk of placental pathology, severe bleeding at delivery and caesarean hysterectomy.[5] Those pregnancies that are more extrinsic to the uterus and approaching the bladder, with little surround-

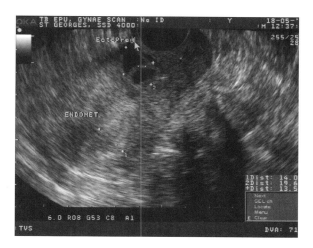

Figure 13.1 Transvaginal scan showing an empty uterus and a gestation sac implanted in the previous Caesarean section scar, bulging anteriorly towards the urinary bladder.

ing myometrium are probably more likely to cause earlier uterine rupture and haemorrhage and therefore need definitive treatment as soon as the diagnosis is made (Table 13.1).

MANAGEMENT

Despite over 90 cases having been described in the literature (Figure 13.1), no standardized treatment protocols have yet been developed for the management of stable women with caesarean scar pregnancies. No one individual method appears to be without potential significant complications.

Initial reports tended to describe surgical management, whereas more recent management usually involves local or systemic methotrexate in the first instance. However, Hasegawa and Chuang have suggested that there may be a reduced chance of recurrence of a scar ectopic in a future pregnancy if surgical resection of the pregnancy and scar has been carried out in the first instance.[33,53] In view of the rare nature of the condition and its threat of serious morbidity and mortality, women with a suspected caesarean scar pregnancy should usually be referred to a specialist centre for confirmation of the diagnosis and management. Massive haemorrhage related to caesarean scar

Table 13.1. Caesarean section scar ectopic pregnancy: reported management methods

Author	Year	No. of cases	Method of management	Comments
Larsen[2]	1978	1	Laparotomy, hysterotomy resection and scar dehiscence repair	
Rempen[12]	1990	1	Laparotomy, hysterotomy, curettage	
Herman[13]	1995	1	Expectant	Diagnosis confirmed at 14 weeks, sac seen bulging into uterine cavity. Uterine rupture and hysterectomy 35/40 (healthy baby)
Lai[14]	1995	1	Methotrexate	Uterine rupture
Ravhon[15]	1997		Systemic methotrexate	
Godin[16]	1997	1	Local potassium chloride and local methotrexate	
Padovan[17]	1998	1	Curettage and systemic methotrexate	
Huang[18]	1998	1	Hysterectomy	Emergency due to severe bleeding
Roberts[19]	1998	1	Local hyperosmolar glucose and systemic methotrexate	
Neiger[20]	1998	1	Attempted suction curettage followed by laparoscopy and laparotomy to resect gestational mass	
Valley[21]	1998	1	Hysterotomy and systemic methotrexate	
Marcus[11]	1999	1	Uterine artery embolization and hysterectomy	Presented at 13/40 with dehiscence and viable pregnancy in scar tissue between uterus and bladder
Lee[22]	1999	1	Hysteroscopy and laparoscopic resection of gestation products	Presented with bleeding 2/52 after attempted termination
Sum[23]	2000	1	Systemic methotrexate and uterine artery embolization	
Seow[24]	2001	1	Laparotomy and local excision of the sac	
Nawroth[25]	2001	1	Systemic and local methotrexate	
Shufaro[26]	2001	1	Systemic methotrexate	
Ayoubi[27]	2001	1	Ultrasound-guided aspiration and systemic methotrexate	
Vial[28]	2001	1	Laparotomy and excision of the gestation mass	
Haimov-Kochman[29]	2002	2	Systemic methotrexate	
Ghezzi[30]	2002	1	Methotrexate, intra-amniotic potassium chloride and uterine artery embolization	
Lam[31]	2002	1	Multiple dose methotrexate and folinic acid	
Fylstra[32]	2002	1	Laparoscopy, laparotomy and hysterotomy	
Imbar[33]	2003	1	Uterine artery embolization	Emergency management after termination attempt for misdiagnosed intrauterine pregnancy
Chuang[34]	2003	1	Local injection of vasopressin, Foley catheter tamponade and systemic methotrexate	Presented as emergency with profuse bleeding
Liang[10]	2003	1	Attempted suction curettage followed by laparotomy and hysterectomy	Emergency management of first trimester uterine rupture and placenta percreta
Yang[35]	2003	3	Uterine artery embolization (2 intra-operative, 1 postoperative)	2 cases with bleeding at attempted termination (misdiagnosed intrauterine), 1 perioperative for misdiagnosed tubal ectopic (this case had laparoscopic resection of gestation mass after)

Author	Year	No. of cases	Method of management	Comments
Hartung[36]	2003	1	Transabdominal local injection of potassium chloride	
Salomon[37]	2003	1	Transvaginal local injection of potassium chloride	6/40 heterotopic. Scar pregnancy injected only. Successful ongoing intrauterine twin, delivered 36/40
Jurkovic[4]	2003	18	8 surgical evacuation (no complications) 7 local methotrexate (5 successful) 3 expectant (1 successful)	5/18 required blood transfusion 1 hysterectomy
Chou[38]	2004	1	Uterine artery embolization	Used 3D colour power Doppler to monitor vascularity before and after procedure
Marchiole[39]	2004	1	Systemic methotrexate, curettage and uterine artery embolization	Haemorrhage at curettage, needing Foley catheter tamponade for 10 days
Seow[3]	2004	12	3 transvaginal injection of methotrexate into embryo/sac 2 transabdominal injection of methotrexate into embryo/sac 2 transabdominal injection followed by systemic 2 systemic methotrexate alone 2 D+C 1 local resection of gestation mass	1 hysterectomy (curettage case) Uterine rupture in 1 woman at 38/40 in subsequent pregnancy
Hsieh[40]	2004	1	Transvaginal embryo aspiration	6/40 IVF triplet pregnancy with 1 sac in scar. Successful outcome for other 2 embryos
Maymon[5]	2004	8	4 methotrexate 1 expectant 1 transvaginal aspiration of sac 2 open surgery	1 term caesarean hysterectomy 1 first trimester hysterotomy and resection of mass (Methotrexate treated group all had uneventful outcome)
Lam[41]	2004	2	Methotrexate	Both cases unsuccessful
Wang[42]	2004	1	Laparoscopic uterine artery ligation and resection of gestational mass	
Arslan[43]	2005	1	Suction curettage	
Tan[44]	2005	2	Local methotrexate	Initial misdiagnosis as miscarriage
Hwu[45]	2005	2	1 Systemic methotrexate followed by TV needle aspiration of the embryo and local methotrexate 1 TV needle aspiration of the embryo and local methotrexate	1 failed methotrexate
Einenkel[46]	2005	1	Emergency hysterectomy	Initial termination of pregnancy attempt as misdiagnosed intrauterine
Sharma[47]	2005	1	Emergency intrauterine Foley catheter, diagnostic laparoscopy, laparotomy and combined abdominal and vaginal suturing	Severe bleeding after failed medical termination of pregnancy and attempted suction termination
Chao[48]	2005	1	Hysteroscopic resection after failed methotrexate and curettage	Resection because of persisting bleeding and hCG levels
Sugawara[49]	2005	3	Uterine artery embolization prior to curettage and methotrexate	
Wang[50]	2005	1	Laparoscopy and resection of gestational contents with suturing of uterus	
Reyftmann[51]	2005	1		Management of massive bleeding in a scar pregnancy
Noguchi[52]	2005	1	Surgical	
Graesslin[53]	2005	1	Systemic methotrexate and curettage	
Ben Nagi[9]	2005	1	Expectant	Placenta praevia and accreta at term necessitating hysterectomy

pregnancies obviously needs emergency surgical procedures, some of which are also described.

SURGICAL MANAGEMENT

Surgical management generally involves either suction curettage or surgical resection of the gestation mass.

Jurkovic described eight surgical evacuations with no serious complications, although three of these women had a blood loss of 500–1000 ml, requiring insertion of a Foley catheter, which was then inflated with up to 90 ml saline to exert pressure on the implantation site to achieve haemostasis.[4] Seow reports two cases of evacuation alone, of which one woman underwent hysterectomy due to profuse vaginal bleeding.[3]

Maymon has used first trimester open hysterotomy to excise the gestation mass with success.[5] Wang has described one case of laparoscopic resection of the gestation mass, with uterine suturing for haemostasis and another case of laparoscopic uterine artery ligation and resection of the gestational mass.[41,49] Seow also treated one patient by surgical resection of the gestation mass.[3]

Marcus used uterine artery embolization and hysterectomy to manage a case where the pregnancy had ruptured through the scar and was located in the scar tissue between the uterus and bladder.[4] Chou employed uterine artery embolization alone, with colour and power Doppler to monitor neovascularization before and after the procedure.[37] Hysteroscopic resection of the gestation sac has also been reported[47].

MEDICAL MANAGEMENT

The folate antagonist methotrexate, either local or systemic, is now the commonest method used to terminate caesarean scar pregnancy. Details of the use of methotrexate are discussed in previous chapters. In his series, Seow described three cases of transvaginal injection of methotrexate into the embryo or sac, four cases of transabdominal injection of methotrexate into the embryo or sac (followed by systemic methotrexate in two of these women) and two cases of systemic methotrexate alone.[3] No significant complications are reported for any of these cases, though time to resolution of the ectopic masses was generally several months. In Maymon's series of eight cases, the four women treated with local and/or systemic methotrexate also had uneventful outcomes.[5]

It seems possible to terminate the pregnancy, however the problem with medical management is that the redundant tissue left behind takes months to resolve and may be associated with persistent discharge and bleeding, or more serious complications. Jurkovic's series describes only five successful outcomes out of seven cases treated with local methotrexate. The two 'failed' cases of medical management required surgical treatment for vaginal bleeding of greater than 1000 ml. Lai also reports a case of rupture after medical treatment and Lam describes the failure of methotrexate in two cases.[4]

Systemic methotrexate may be given as a one-off dose, usually in the region of 50 mg/m^2. Further doses may be given at an interval of several days, if the pregnancy fails to regress. Alternate-day methotrexate and 'rescue' folinic acid has also been effective.

Transvaginal or transabdominal potassium chloride injection into the sac or embryo has been used successfully, one such case being a heterotopic pregnancy where the remaining intrauterine gestation continued successfully to 36 weeks.[36] However, potassium chloride alone, though it usually causes embryonic demise, may be insufficient to prevent further trophoblast proliferation and has therefore generally been used in combination with other techniques, such as methotrexate.[16,30] Jurkovic reports another heterotopic pregnancy, and describes the local injection of the scar pregnancy with potassium chloride, and the coexisting intrauterine twin continuing to 31 weeks when emergency caesarean section was performed for antepartum haemorrhage, possibly related to the deficient uterine scar.[4] A further heterotopic pregnancy in a caesarean scar has been treated successfully with transvaginal aspiration of the embryo, with successful delivery of the other two of the original IVF triplets.[39]

The follow-up time is variable after methotrexate treatment, with serum hCG usually taking several weeks to return to non-pregnant values, and ultrasound appearances of the residual mass lasting as long as 1 year.[1,3,29] This requires patient compliance, with at least weekly follow up initially, though the frequency of visits can be reduced once the pregnancy has been shown to be regressing.

Combination management

Dilatation and curettage followed by systemic methotrexate, uterine artery embolization prior to curettage and methotrexate, hysteroscopic resection after failed methotrexate and curettage, systemic methotrexate and curettage, methotrexate, intra-amniotic potassium chloride and uterine artery embolization, hysterotomy and systemic methotrexate are some of the combined medical and surgical approaches which have been used.[17,21,30,37,52]

Emergency management

Women with profuse bleeding, either intra-abdominal or vaginal, from a disrupted or ruptured caesarean scar pregnancy need immediate surgical management. This may involve laparotomy and hysterectomy though uterine artery embolization or ligation has been successful intraoperatively, postoperatively and in some cases preoperatively in several reports.[11,18,32,34,45]

FUTURE PREGNANCIES

Although a case of a repeat caesarean scar pregnancy has been reported, many authors have reported normally implanted intrauterine pregnancies after successful treatment of a caesarean scar pregnancy.[3,4,53] However, the risk remains of severe complications. In Seow's series of eight cases, one maternal and fetal death occurred due to uterine rupture at 38 weeks in a subsequent pregnancy after prior treatment of a caesarean scar pregnancy with suction curettage and Foley catheter tamponade. He recommends an interval of at least 3 months and preferably 1–2 years after a

caesarean scar pregnancy to reduce the chance of further complications. He also suggests early elective caesarean section to minimize the chance of uterine rupture near term.[3]

A PROPOSED MANAGEMENT STRATEGY

As the available evidence does not favour any one particular mode of treatment for caesarean scar pregnancies, the decision regarding treatment must be made on the basis of gestation, pregnancy viability, myometrial integrity, clinical symptoms and informed discussion with the woman herself.[4] Furthermore a lack of clarity in relation to the natural history of this condition renders an evidence-based approach to this condition very difficult. In general, however, because of the risk of massive haemorrhage if the pregnancy progresses to term, most authors strongly recommend termination of the pregnancy in the first trimester for all caesarean scar pregnancies.[44]

In our unit we have generally used medical management (local or systemic methotrexate) for the haemodynamically stable woman diagnosed with a caesarean scar pregnancy, after careful counselling. Recently, however, we have successfully managed two women (with viable 6 and 8 week caesarean scar pregnancies) with a new strategy, combining systemic methotrexate ($50 \, mg/m^2$) to achieve pregnancy regression, followed by semielective ultrasound-guided suction curettage once colour Doppler imaging has confirmed minimal residual vascularity. In this way, the gestational mass could be removed, but only once the vascularity of the implantation site had significantly reduced, thus minimizing the operative risk. Both women had normal serum βhCG levels within 5 weeks of initial presentation and methotrexate injection. One of the women was managed as an outpatient, though the second was admitted for social reasons. Neither experienced any complications and specifically had no significant blood loss and preserved their fertility.

This management strategy can be undertaken if the clinical condition is stable and the patient is compliant. The woman needs to have 24-hour access to a member of the early pregnancy or gynaecology team and be aware to attend the hospital if there are any signs of significant pain or bleeding. Full blood count, liver function and renal function need to be taken and repeated after 7 days to check for complications of methotrexate treatment.

After the first dose of methotrexate, if the serum hCG is falling, then a second dose is given around day 5. If the serum hCG is not declining then aspiration of the sac and direct injection of 25 mg methotrexate is considered.

The suction curettage is performed by a senior gynaecologist, with initial insertion of the curette facing posteriorly to minimize uncontrolled trauma to the myometrial area in the region of the caesarean section scar. The curette is then rotated anteriorly and suction started in order to aspirate the sac in a controlled fashion under ultrasound guidance. Laparoscopy and laparotomy equipment are immediately available, should intraperitoneal bleeding occur and the need for resection of the scar arise. Cross-matched blood is also available in case of perioperative haemorrhage.

Serum hCG follow up is continued weekly until the hCG falls below 15 IU/L.

In the haemodynamically compromised woman, clearly this protocol is not appropriate and the woman needs immediate surgery, with availability of suction curettage (preferably ultrasound-guided) and tamponade in the form of a large Foley catheter or Cook's intrauterine catheter. It is necessary to have equipment to perform laparoscopy to assess for intraperitoneal haemorrhage and perform laparoscopic or open resection of the sac and scar if indicated. Uterine artery ligation or embolization, or hysterectomy may also be useful in cases of massive haemorrhage to save the life of the woman.

It must be emphasized that this is one approach to the management of this difficult condition. However there appears to be a growing consensus that destroying the trophoblast in isolation is not sufficient, and that the pregnancy has to be removed as part of the management. Debate centres in relation to how and when this should be done.

Advising women regarding future pregnancy is largely based on anecdotal evidence and we do not know if it would be of benefit to revise a woman's caesarean section scar before embarking on a future pregnancy. It seems sensible to try to direct these cases towards specialist centres both to improve the outcome for patients and also in order to gather sufficient data to formulate evidence-based guidelines. It is likely this will take some time, particularly in relation to safety data.

CASE REPORT

A 30-year-old woman presented to the Early Pregnancy Unit complaining of vaginal bleeding for 5 hours. She had a positive pregnancy test, with a gestational age of 6 weeks and 1 day by certain menstrual dates. Her previous obstetric history included three caesarean sections (two living children, one stillbirth) and one miscarriage.

At her first assessment no obvious gestation sac was visible on transvaginal ultrasound but a thickened endometrium of 12.2 mm was noted. No free fluid or adnexal masses were detected. The differential diagnosis of a failed pregnancy or a scar pregnancy was made.

Initial serum hCG was 6000 IU/L and a repeat scan was performed that day (day 1) by a senior doctor in the department, at which time a small gestational sac was noted in the region of the internal os, with prominent high-velocity, low-impedance blood flow on Doppler examination.

The woman was admitted because she spoke very little English and therefore we could not be confident that she could adequately understand the implications of the diagnosis or advice about outpatient management.

Intramuscular methotrexate (50 mg/m²) was given on day 4 after a further scan supported the diagnosis of a scar pregnancy. Repeat scan on day 6 showed that the pregnancy was indeed viable as a fetal pole and heartbeat were visible. The hCG was 12769 IU/L, but fell to 10673 IU/L by day 8. At this point a second dose of methotrexate was given.

The heartbeat was no longer visible on day 10 and a steady decline in vascularity of the sac and fall in hCG followed. On day 21 ultrasound-guided suction curettage was performed under general anaesthetic by a senior operator, with cross-matched blood immediately available as well as equipment for possible laparoscopy or laparotomy. However the procedure was uneventful, with less than 500 ml blood loss. The patient was discharged the following day, with regular outpatient βhCG follow up until the βhCG fell to 4 IU/L (day 35).

PRACTICAL POINTS

1. With the increasing incidence of caesarean section and apparent increase in scar pregnancies, all women with previous caesarean section who undergo assessment for early pregnancy pain or bleeding should be carefully examined to exclude a caesarean scar pregnancy.
2. Women with a suspected caesarean scar pregnancy should be referred immediately to a specialist centre for confirmation of the diagnosis and appropriate treatment.
3. No one management strategy is without risk or complications and the treatment decision should be based on gestation, pregnancy viability, myometrial integrity, clinical symptoms, likely compliance with medical management and informed discussion with the woman herself.
4. Evidence at present does not support a role for expectant management.
5. Initial management with local or systemic methotrexate, often in repeated doses, is the commonest treatment strategy, and can be combined with suction curettage of the gestation mass once vascularity has diminished.
6. Women with significant bleeding or haemodynamic compromise need immediate surgical management, and should be counselled about the risk of hysterectomy.

REFERENCES

1. Fylstra DL. Ectopic pregnancy within a cesarean scar: a review. Obstet Gynecol Surv 2002; 57:537–43.
2. Larsen JV, Solomon MH. Pregnancy in a uterine scar sacculus- An unusual case of postabortal haemorrhage. A case report. S Afr Med J 1978; 28:142–3.
3. Seow KM, Huang LW, Lin YH, et al. Cesarean scar pregnancy: issues in management. Ultrasound Obstet Gynecol 2004; 23:247–53.
4. Jurkovic D, Hillaby K, Woelfer B, et al. First-trimester diagnosis and management of pregnancies implanted into the lower uterine segment Cesarean section scar. Ultrasound Obstet Gynecol 2003; 21:310.
5. Maymon R, Halperin R, Mendlovic S, et al. Ectopic pregnancies in a Caesarean scar: review of the medical approach to an iatrogenic complication. Hum Reprod 2004; 19(2):278–84.
6. Hemminki E, Merilainen J. Long-term effects of cesarean sections: ectopic pregnancies and placental problems. Am J Obstet Gynecol 1996; 174:1569–74.
7. Fabunmi L, Perks N. Caesarean section scar ectopic pregnancy following postcoital contraception. J Fam Plann Reprod Health Care 2002; 28(3):155–6.
8. Shih JC. Cesarean scar pregnancy: diagnosis with three-dimensional (3D) ultrasound and 3D power Doppler. Ultrasound Obstet Gynecol 2004; 23(3):306–7.
9. Ben Nagi J, Ofili-Yebovi D, Marsh M, Jurkovic D. First-trimester cesarean scar pregnancy evolving into placenta previa/accreta at term. J Ultrasound Med 2005; 24:1569–73.
10. Liang HS, Jeng CJ, Sheen TC, et al. First-trimester uterine rupture from a placenta percreta. A case report. J Reprod Med 2003; 48(6):474–8.
11. Marcus S, Cheng E, Goff B. Extrauterine pregnancy resulting from early uterine rupture. Obstet Gynecol 1999; 94:804–5.
12. Rempen A, Albert P. Diagnosis and therapy of an ectopic in the cesarean section scar implanted early pregnancy]. Z Geburtsh u Perinat 1990; 194:46–8.
13. Herman A, Weinraub Z, Avrech O, et al. Follow up and outcome of isthmic pregnancy located in a previous caesarean section scar. Br J Obstet Gynaecol 1995; 102:839–41.
14. Lai YM, Lee JD, Lee CL, Chen TC, Soong YK. An ectopic pregnancy embedded in the myometrium of a previous cesarean section scar. Acta Obstet Gynecol Scand 1995; 74:573–6.
15. Ravhon A, Ben-Chetrit A, Rabinowitz R, Neuman M, Beller U. Successful methotrexate treatment of a viable pregnancy within a thin uterine scar. BJOG 1997; 104:628–9.

16. Godin PA, Bassil S, Donnez J. An ectopic pregnancy developing in a previous caesarian section scar. Fertil Steril 1997; 67:398–400.

17. Padovan P, Lauri F, Marchetti M. Intrauterine ectopic pregnancy. A case report. Clin Exp Obstet Gynecol 1998; 25:79–80.

18. Huang KH, Lee CL, Wang CJ, Soong YK, Lee KF. Pregnancy in a previous cesarean section scar: case report. Changgeng Yi Xue Za Zhi 1998; 21:323–7.

19. Roberts H, Kohlenber C, Lanzarone V, Murray H. Ectopic pregnancy in lower segment uterine scar. Aust NZ J Obstet Gynecol 1998; 38:114–16.

20. Neiger R, Weldon K, Means N. Intramural pregnancy in a cesarean section scar. A case report. J Reprod Med 1998; 43(11):999–1001.

21. Valley MT, Pierce JG, Daniel TB, Kaunitz AM. Cesarean scar pregnancy: imaging and treatment with conservative surgery. Obstet Gynecol 1998; 91:838–40.

22. Lee CL, Wang CJ, Chao A, Yen CF, Soong YK. Laparoscopic management of an ectopic pregnancy in a previous Caesarean section scar. Hum Reprod 1999; 14:1234–6.

23. Sum TK, Wong SH, Tai CM, Ng TK. An ectopic pregnancy in a previous caesarean section scar: treatment with systemic methotrexate and uterine artery embolisation. J Obstet Gynaecol 2000; 20:328.

24. Seow KM, Hwang JL, Tsai YL. Ultrasound diagnosis of a pregnancy in a Cesarean section scar. Ultrasound Obstet Gynecol 2001; 18:547–9.

25. Nawroth F, Foth D, Wilhelm L, et al. Conservative treatment of ectopic pregnancy in a cesarean section scar with methotrexate: a case report. Eur J Obstet Gynecol Reprod Biol 2001; 99:135–7.

26. Shufaro Y, Nadjari M. Implantation of a gestational sac in a cesarean section scar. Fertil Steril 2001; 75:1217.

27. Ayoubi JM, Fanchin R, Meddoun M, Fernandez H, Pons JC. Conservative treatment of complicated cesarean scar pregnancy. Acta Obstet Gynecol Scand 2001; 80:469–70.

28. Vial Y, Petignat P, Hohlfeld P. Pregnancy in a cesarean scar. Ultrasound Obstet Gynecol 2000; 16:592–3.

29. Haimov-Kochman R, Sciaky-Tamir Y, Yanai N, Yagel S. Conservative management of two ectopic pregnancies implanted in previous uterine scars. Ultrasound Obstet Gynecol 2002; 19:616–9.

30. Ghezzi F, Lagana D, Franchi M, Fugazzola C, Bolis P. Conservative treatment by chemotherapy and uterine arteries embolization of a cesarean scar pregnancy. Eur J Obstet Gynecol Reprod Biol 2002; 103:88–91.

31. Lam PM, Lo KW. Multiple-dose methotrexate for pregnancy in a cesarean section scar. A case report. J Reprod Med 2002; 47:332–4.

32. Fylstra DL, Pound-Chang T, Miller MG, Cooper A, Miller KM. Ectopic pregnancy within a cesarean delivery scar: a case report. Am J Obstet Gynecol 2002; 187:302–4.

33. Imbar T, Bloom A, Ushakov F, Yagel S. Uterine artery embolization to control hemorrhage after termination of pregnancy implanted in a cesarean delivery scar. J Ultrasound Me. 2003; 22:1111–5.

34. Chuang J, Seow KM, Cheng WC, Tsai YL, Hwang JL. Conservative treatment of ectopic pregnancy in a caesarean section scar. BJOG 2003; 110:869–70.

35. Yang MJ, Jeng MH. Combination of transarterial embolization of uterine arteries and conservative surgical treatment for pregnancy in a cesarean section scar. A report of 3 cases. J Reprod Med 2003; 48:213–6.

36. Hartung J, Meckies J. Management of a case of uterine scar pregnancy by transabdominal potassium chloride injection. Ultrasound Obstet Gynecol 2003; 21:94–5.

37. Salomon LJ, Fernandez H, Chauveaud A, Doumerc S, Frydman R. Successful management of a heterotopic Caesarean scar pregnancy: potassium chloride injection with preservation of the intrauterine gestation: case report. Hum Reprod 2003; 18:189–91.

38. Chou MM, Hwang JI, Tseng JJ, Huang YF, Ho ES. Cesarean scar pregnancy: quantitative assessment of uterine neovascularization with 3-dimensional color power Doppler imaging and successful treatment with uterine artery embolisation. Am J Obstet Gynecol 2004; 190:866–8.

39. Marchiole P, Gorlero F, de Caro G, Podesta M, Valenzano M. Intramural pregnancy embedded in a previous Cesarean section scar treated conservatively. Ultrasound Obstet Gynecol 2004; 23:307–9.

40. Hsieh BC, Hwang JL, Pan HS, et al. Heterotopic Caesarean scar pregnancy combined with intrauterine pregnancy successfully treated with embryo aspiration for selective embryo reduction: case report. Hum Reprod 2004; 19:285–7.

41. Lam PM, Lo KW, Lau TK. Unsuccessful medical treatment of cesarean scar ectopic pregnancy with systemic methotrexate: a report of two cases. Acta Obstet Gynecol Scand 2004; 83:108–11.

42. Wang CJ, Yuen LT, Yen CF, Lee CL, Soong YK. Three-dimensional power Doppler ultrasound diagnosis and laparoscopic management of a pregancy in a previous cesarean scar. J Laparoendosc Adv Surg Tech A 2004; 14:399–402.

43. Arslan M, Pata O, Dilek TU, et al. Treatment of viable cesarean scar ectopic pregnancy with suction curettage. Int J Gynaecol Obstet 2005; 89:163–6.

44. Tan G, Chong YS, Biswas A. Caesarean scar pregnancy: a diagnosis to consider carefully in patients with risk factors. Ann Acad Med Singapore 2005; 34:216–9.

45. Hwu YM, Hsu CY, Yang HY. Conservative treatment of caesarean scar pregnancy with transvaginal needle aspiration of the embryo. BJOG 2005; 112:841–842.

46. Einenkel J, Stumpp P, Kosling S, Horn LC, Hockel M. A misdiagnosed case of caesarean scar pregnancy. Arch Gynecol Obstet 2005; 271:178–81.

47. Sharma S, Imoh-Ita F. Surgical management of caesarean scar pregnancy. J Obstet Gynaecol 2005; 25:525–6.

48. Chao A, Wang TH, Wang CJ, Lee CL, Chao AS. Hysteroscopic management of cesarean scar pregnancy after unsuccessful methotrexate treatment. J Minim Invasive Gynecol 2005; 12:374–6.

49. Sugawara J, Senoo M, Chisaka H, Yaegashi N, Okamura K. Successful conservative treatment of a cesarean scar pregnancy with uterine artery embolization. Tohoku J Exp Med 2005; 206:261–5.

50. Wang YL, Su TH, Chen HS. Laparoscopic management of an ectopic pregnancy in a lower segment cesarean section scar: a review and case report. J Minim Invasive Gynecol 2005; 12:73–9.

51. Reyftmann L, Vernhet H, Boulot P. Management of massive uterine bleeding in a cesarean scar pregnancy. Int J Gynaecol Obstet 2005; 89:154–5.

52. Noguchi S, Adachi M, Konishi H, et al. Intramural pregnancy in a previous cesarean section scar: a case report on conservative surgery. Acta Obstet Gynecol Scand 2005; 84:493–5.

53. Graesslin O, Dedecker F Jr, Quereux C, Gabriel R. Conservative treatment of ectopic pregnancy in a cesarean scar. Obstet Gynecol 2005; 105:869–71.

54. Hasegawa J, Ichizuka K, Matsuoka R, et al. Limitations of conservative treatment for repeat Cesarean scar pregnancy. Ultrasound Obstet Gynecol 2005; 25:310–1.

EDITORIAL COMMENT

We have seen how to manage the clinical situation where a pregnancy cannot be seen anywhere in the pelvis in the presence of a positive pregnancy test. At one time this invariably led to a laparoscopy to exclude an ectopic pregnancy. We now label these women as having a pregnancy of unknown location (PUL). How these patients are managed depends on the quality of the ultrasound service that is available. An indicator of quality is the prevalence of PULs in the early pregnancy population. A further indication is the number of ectopic pregnancies in the PUL group. The better the scanning, the more early intrauterine and ectopic pregnancies will be seen, hence the number of ectopic pregnancies seen in the PUL population will be low (10–15%). These are reasonable benchmarks against which an early pregnancy unit can be judged. However we must be realistic. We have seen that in good quality scanning units the use of discriminatory zones is not helpful, however in some units they will be, as a number of large ectopic pregnancies will be missed on ultrasound.

It is clear that the management of ectopic pregnancy has changed significantly. Laparoscopy was once the standard for diagnosis. This is no longer the case. We have seen how with adequate training over 90% of tubal ectopic pregnancies will be visualized with vaginal ultrasonography. Earlier diagnosis has opened up the possibility of more conservative management strategies. Clinically we now see more ectopic pregnancies that have either minimal or no symptoms. As a result treatment now emphasizes reduced intervention and the retention of potential fertility.

Like miscarriage, ectopic pregnancy used to invariably be seen as a surgical emergency and a laparotomy was the likely outcome. This is still the case in some instances, but it is certainly not the usual outcome. If surgery is performed it is likely to be laparoscopic and involve a salpingostomy with preservation of the affected tube. There is also a recognition that a number of ectopic pregnancies will resolve without intervention, and in an increasing number of cases we can now adopt a watch-and-wait

approach. Patient selection is vital in these cases. In general a relatively low initial hCG and progesterone are associated with a resolving pregnancy that does not require intervention. By waiting for the trend in hCG over time to be established we can improve on this approach. Even with a relatively high initial hCG if the hCG ratio is low, then expectant management if likely to be a good option. Conversely as the hCG ratio increases the likelihood of needing methotrexate increases. In this way giving unnecessary methotrexate can be avoided.

When treating women with methotrexate the existing algorithms seem to predict a successful outcome with a reasonable degree of accuracy. Managing ectopic pregnancies conservatively is not without risk, and patients must be made aware of this. Compliance is essential and there must be a facility for patients to contact a clinician at any time if they develop pain or need to be reviewed. Nevertheless there are not a great deal of safety data in the literature with respect to this approach to management and caution is advised if there are any doubts about either patient compliance, follow up arrangements or the clinical situation.

Surgery for ectopic pregnancy is now carried out laparoscopically in by far the majority of cases. Training is an issue, however any unit that deals with early pregnancy complication should have access to a surgeon who is competent to deal with these problems. For stable early ectopic pregnancies this surgery is not an emergency. It can be scheduled as a day surgical procedure within a day or so of diagnosis.

Non-tubal ectopic pregnancies represent a particular challenge. For cornual pregnancies it seems clear that for the majority, methotrexate will be successful. For cervical and in particular for section scar ectopic pregnancies the situation is less clear. The common thread is that if an embryo is present, it must be terminated. However the problem is what to do next. A consensus seems to be forming that the pregnancy then needs to be removed surgically – the timing of this and whether adjunctive medical treatment should also be given is a matter for debate. The rising rate of caesarean sections in many countries makes this a problem that is likely to become more significant in the future.

We must not be complacent. Ectopic pregnancies can rupture unpredictably. Furthermore, in many parts of the world discussing the finer points of hCG ratios and methotrexate must seem fatuous. We must remember that for many women ectopic pregnancy remains a life-threatening condition. Even in the UK it remains a significant cause of death. Simply providing urinary pregnancy tests for women with pelvic pain would reduce some of the damage. Solutions do not have to be complicated to be effective.

Finally we must pay attention to prevention. The evidence linking *Chlamydia* infection and ectopic pregnancy is convincing. Appropriately directed screening and enhanced awareness of this condition may make an impact.

14

The diagnosis and management of trophoblastic tumours in early pregnancy

Eric Jauniaux and Michael J Seckl

Introduction • Pathophysiology of complete and partial hydatidiform moles • Clinical and ultrasound diagnosis of GTD in early pregnancy • Conclusions • Practical points

INTRODUCTION

Gestational trophoblastic disease (GTD) is a term that incorporates a wide spectrum of disorders of trophoblast development, ranging from hydatidiform mole at the benign end to malignant choriocarcinoma. The most common GTD are complete and partial hydatidiform moles (PHM). The estimated incidence of partial mole is 1 per 700 pregnancies whereas the incidence of complete mole is around 1 per 1500–2000 pregnancies.[1–3]

Both complete and partial molar pregnancies are associated with persistent trophoblastic disease and are offered follow up to ensure complete disappearance of trophoblastic tissue. Following uterine evacuation about 10–20% of women with a complete mole develop persistent GTD (pGTD).[2] The incidence of this complication after a partial mole varies widely between 0.1 and 11%,[1–6] probably due to the absence of epidemiological data on large unselected populations. Difficulties lie in the diagnosis of both CHM and PHM in early pregnancy because both ultrasound and histological appearances differ between the first and second trimester and cases can be missed.

The vast majority of complete and partial moles miscarry spontaneously during the first 3–4 months of pregnancy resulting in an incidence of molar placenta of 1 per 41 miscarriages.[3] These data suggest that most women with GTD are likely to be first seen in an Early Pregnancy Unit (EPU) and an accurate diagnosis is thus essential to optimize the management of these women. The antenatal ultrasound diagnosis of complete mole usually poses little problem from the third month of pregnancy onwards and can be made antenatally in around 80% of the cases (Figure 14.1).[7–12] By

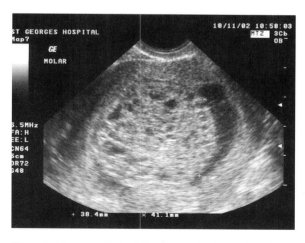

Figure 14.1 Complete hydatidiform mole. (Reproduced from G. Condous. The management of early pregnancy complications. Best Pract Res Clin Obstet Gynaecol. 2004;18:37–57, with permission from Elsevier.)

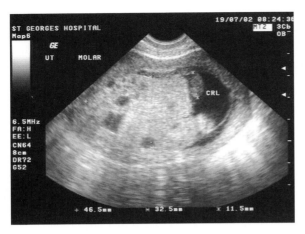

Figure 14.2 Partial hydatidiform mole. (Reproduced from G. Condous. The management of early pregnancy complications. Best Pract Res Clin Obstet Gynaecol. 2004;18:37–57, with permission from Elsevier.)

contrast, the ultrasound diagnosis of partial mole is less accurate and around 70% of those cases will be missed antenatally (Figure 14.2).[8-12] There is a clear advantage for the women to be informed about the diagnosis of GTD as quickly as possible so that an adequate follow up can be initiated. The aim of this chapter is to describe the early diagnosis and management of GTD detected in an early pregnancy unit.

PATHOPHYSIOLOGY OF COMPLETE AND PARTIAL HYDATIDIFORM MOLES

The distinction between complete and partial mole was made in the late 1970s on the basis of gross morphological, histological and cytogenetic criteria.[13,14] The clinical and pathological picture of the two molar syndromes overlap to a degree since both the phenotype and natural history of the partial mole seem to represent a mild, bland version of those of the complete mole.

Complete or classical hydatidiform moles (CHM)

These correspond to a generalized swelling of the villous tissue, diffuse trophoblastic hyperplasia and no embryonic or fetal tissue.

Complete moles are diploid with chromosomes totally derived from the paternal genome probably resulting from the fertilization of an 'empty oocyte', devoid of the maternal X,23 by a single spermatozoon whose chromosomes double without cell cytokinesis.[17] This totally androgenic conceptus is characterized by generalized trophoblastic hyperplasia and rapidly developing villous oedema with central cistern formation, giving the macroscopic appearance of a 'bunch of grapes'. The fluid, at first uniformly distributed in the core of the villi, collects in several loculi to coalesce into a central cistern.[15-17]

Partial hydatidiform mole (PHM)

This term refers to the combination of a fetus with localized placental molar degenerations. Histologically it is characterized by focal swelling of the villous tissue, focal trophoblastic hyperplasia and embryonic or fetal tissue.[13-15] The abnormal villi are scattered within macroscopically normal placental tissue that tends to retain its shape. Theoretically, the histopathological definition should only be applied when villous hydatiform changes are associated with trophoblastic hyperplasia, which cannot be demonstrated by ultrasound. The hydatidiform changes are also focal resulting in an irregular patchwork of seemingly normal and affected areas. Digynic triploidies occasionally show an irregular contour and a mild form of trophoblastic hyperplasia.[18] Thus diagnostic errors may be caused by unusually conspicuous trophoblastic anomalies but also to insufficient placental sampling. The sensitivity and specificity of microscopic examination in these cases can be improved to reach 70% by adding features of the materno–embryonic interface to classical villous histological criteria.[19]

Partial moles are in about 90% of the cases triploid, having inherited two sets of chromosomes from the father and one from the mother.[21,22] Two fetal phenotypes have been delineated: type I (paternally derived, i.e. diandric triploidy) fetuses are relatively well-grown, have a proportionate head size and are associated with placental partial molar changes; in type II (maternally derived, i.e. digynic triploidy) fetuses present with severe asymmetrical growth restriction and an apparently normal placenta.[21,22]

Early cytogenetic studies have suggested that the majority of triploidies are of diandric origin, resulting from the fertilization of a haploid ovum either by two single sperms or a single diploid sperm.[15,23] Less than one-third of triploidies encountered in the first trimester are of digynic origin resulting from a double maternal haploid contribution when the ovum fails to undergo the first or second meiotic division before fertilization.[23] Triploid diandric partial moles are certainly more common in EPL than non-molar digynic triploidies[24] but seem to be associated with a lower risk of pGTD than second-trimester triploid partial moles.[25]

Pathophysiology of villous hydatidiform transformation

The biochemical analysis of the molar fluid suggests that it is derived from diffusion of the maternal plasma and/or by synthesis by the trophoblast and that in the case of PHM it is unchanged by any fetal metabolism.[26] Thus hydropic (hydatidiform) transformation of the villous mesenchyme results from a lack, maldevelopment or regression of the villous vasculature that makes the drainage of fluid supplied by the trophoblast impossible. Mild-to-moderate generalized villous oedema can follow the demise of an embryo or early fetus. However, gross waterlogging and villous cistern formation is found only in CHM and PHM. Finally, although there is a well-established clinical association between molar changes of the villi and trophoblastic hyperplasia, hydropic villous changes can be found in conditions unrelated to gestational trophoblastic disorders (GTD).

Routine histological examination of products of conception

Routine histopathological examination in sporadic miscarriage has generated a great deal of debate and controversy mainly because of the inaccuracy of histological criteria in identifying the cause of an early pregnancy failure.[27–29] As we have heard in earlier chapters

it is well established that more than 50% of sporadic miscarriages are associated with a chromosomal defect of the conceptus and that the incidence of a chromosomal abnormality increases with increasing maternal age and decreasing gestational age.[29] Most of these abnormalities are numerical chromosomal abnormalities and less than 10% are caused by structural abnormalities or other genetic mechanisms. The overall recurrence risk of numerical chromosomal abnormalities is low and the risk of liveborn trisomy following an aneuploid early pregnancy failure is around 1%.[29] Within this context the role of routine histology for sporadic miscarriage is limited, however its relevance lies in the fact that molar pregnancy is a condition which needs to be detected because of the potential long-term risk of pGTD.[30,31]

CLINICAL AND ULTRASOUND DIAGNOSIS OF GTD IN EARLY PREGNANCY

Ultrasonographic examination of the placenta should correctly identify vesicular villi by the beginning of the second trimester.[10,17,32] Before 13 weeks' gestation some partial moles may present as an enlarged placenta without or with only a few vesicular changes.[33] Since the introduction of early ultrasonography the classification of molar pregnancies has become more difficult because they are evacuated earlier and before the stage of development at which they have the classical morphological features.

Singleton CHM

Classically, women with singleton CHM present with vaginal bleeding, uterine enlargement greater than expected for gestational age and abnormally high levels of serum human chorionic gonadotrophin (hCG). Medical complications include pregnancy-induced hypertension (PIH), hyperthyroidism, hyperemesis, anaemia and the development of ovarian theca lutein cysts. The ovarian hyperstimulation and enlargement of both ovaries may subsequently lead to ovarian torsion or rupture of theca lutein cysts. Now that earlier diagnosis is more common, the incidence of

Table 14.1. Ultrasound differential diagnosis of molar GTD and pGTD in early pregnancy	
Category	Ultrasound features
Complete hydatidiform mole (CHM)	
Single CHM	Avascular snowstorm appearance
	No fetus/multicystic ovaries
Twin/triplet CHM	Avascular snowstorm appearance
	Multicystic ovaries
	Normal fetus with normal placenta
Partial hydatidiform mole (PHM)	
On-going pregnancy	Swiss cheese appearance/placentomegaly
	Small CRL (<10th centile)
	Fetal malformation (rare <12 weeks)
Miscarriages	Increased gestational sac diameter ratios
	Cystic changes in the placenta
	Increased placental echogenicity
Persistent trophoblastic disease	
	Hypoechoic areas (lacunae) surrounded by irregular echogenic areas (trophoblastic nodules) and numerous intramyometrial signals (vascular shunts)
	Low resistance to flow and high peak systolic velocity in the uterine and intratumoral vessels

these complications has decreased.[2] Molar changes can now be detected from the second month of pregnancy by ultrasound which typically reveals a uterine cavity filled with multiple sonolucent areas of varying size and shape ('snowstorm appearance') without any associated embryonic or fetal structures (Figure 14.1). Large sonolucent areas or maternal lakes due to stasis of maternal blood in between the molar villi are often found.[32] Theca lutein cysts secondary to the very high hCG levels may be diagnosed in up to 30% of the cases producing enlarged ovaries with either a 'soap bubble' or 'spoke wheel' appearance.[32] The role of Doppler is limited, although it almost always demonstrates high velocities and low resistance to flow in the uterine arterial circulation and will only be of clinical interest in the diagnosis of an invasive mole.[32]

Usually, the ultrasonographic description of CHM applies to pregnancies between 9 and 12 weeks of amenorrhoea (Table 14.1). Prior to this, demonstrating villous hydatidiform changes using ultrasound may be very difficult and inaccurate.[32] Uterine dysgerminomas, which are the most frequent malignant germ cell tumour in women, may appear as a heterogeneous intrauterine mass with multiple echolucent spaces. Other uterine tumours such as sarcomas or lymphomas may also have features similar to those of a CHM on ultrasound and should theoretically be considered in the differential diagnosis.[32] These tumours do not usually produce hormonal tumour markers such as hCG or alpha-fetoprotein (AFP). Within the context of an early pregnancy failure, previous ultrasound data[7–11] and our recent series comparing ultrasound and histological features[12] indicate that at least 80% of CHM should be diagnosed at the time of the first ultrasound examination. As ongoing CHM are associated with beta hCG levels of 10–200 MoM (multiples of the median), and PHM with levels of 10–60 MoM,[7,11,34] pre-evacuation hCG levels may be a useful adjunct to histology in first-trimester spontaneous miscarriages. This is particularly so in cases with unusual ultrasound appearances.

CHM in multiple pregnancies

A classical mole may coexist with a normal fetus and placenta in cases of molar transformation of one ovum in a dizygotic twin pregnancy. This rare condition has been most frequently diagnosed at around 15–20 weeks, a later gestational age than would be expected with a complete mole. We have found that as a complete mole produces a characteristic vesicular sonographic pattern, their association with a normal gestational sac can be accurately determined at around 12–14 weeks.[7,32] The incidence of GTD in the first trimester of pregnancy is unknown but as vaginal bleeding is the most common presenting symptom (in 96% of the cases), the first ultrasound examination for these women is likely to take place in the Early Pregnancy Unit. An early ultrasound diagnosis may be difficult, because the molar placenta may partially cover the normal placenta. The ultrasound diagnosis becomes easier as pregnancy advances as the marked generalized swelling of the molar tissue with large haemorrhagic areas can be more easily identified on ultrasound. The mother must be informed that if she wishes to continue the pregnancy she will be at high risk of developing severe medical complications classically described in CHM and in particular pre-eclampsia (47%) but also premature delivery and intrauterine fetal death.[7,11] This type of GTD is associated with very high maternal serum hCG levels[34] which can be used to monitor the growth of the molar mass in women deciding to continue with the pregnancy until fetal viability is reached.

Polyploid PHM

Vaginal bleeding in the first or second trimester with a total incidence of 47% is the most common maternal symptom reported in both types of triploidies (Table 14.1). The phenotypic expression of both diandric and digynic triploidies includes growth restriction and disturbance of organogenesis that becomes obvious in fetuses surviving into the second trimester. From 16 weeks, almost all triploid fetuses have a least one measurement below the normal range and more than 70% present with severe growth restriction.[7,32,33] It must be highlighted that more than 80% of fetuses with a triploid partial mole (diandric) present with symmetrical growth restriction, which is important from a differential diagnosis point of view. In these cases, abnormal umbilical artery flow velocity waveforms have been reported as early as 12 weeks of gestation[35] and the fetus may already appear growth restricted with crown–rump length measurements below the 10th centile for gestational age.[32,33] Structural fetal defects are observed antenatally in about 93% of all the cases.[7,32,33] The most common are abnormalities of the hands, bilateral cerebral ventriculomegaly, heart anomalies and micrognathia but these cannot be routinely diagnosed in the first trimester of pregnancy.

As triploidy is a highly lethal chromosomal abnormality, most embryos affected by this defect will die within a few weeks following conception and thus women with partial moles will be first seen by the early pregnancy unit team. In PHM, the hydatidiform transformation is slower and before 12 weeks' gestation some partial mole may present as an enlarged placenta without obvious macroscopic vesicular changes.[7,32,33] It is therefore not surprising that the ultrasound diagnosis of partial mole is less accurate and around 70% of those cases will be missed antenatally.[8] In our recent series,[12] of the 18 cases that were not detected prior to evacuation, 17 (95%) were PHM. Until recently up to 50% of women with complete moles miscarried spontaneously before the diagnosis was made. Several ultrasound features have been proposed that might increase the ultrasound detection of molar change in missed miscarriages in the first trimester. These include gestational sac diameter ratios, cystic changes in the placenta and the increased echogenicity of placental tissue.[8,12,36,37]

As mentioned before, pre-evacuation hCG levels may be a useful adjunct to histology in first-trimester spontaneous miscarriages, in particular in cases with unusual ultrasound appearances.[12] Nine of our 13 molar pregnancies in which a preoperative hCG was available demonstrated an hCG of 2–10.8 MoM. Karyotype or ploidy determination could also be useful in the diagnosis of difficult cases, but are not useful as first-line diagnostic tools as they are expensive and time consuming. DNA ploidy can be useful in problem cases to discriminate between PHM and CHM and is cheaper and faster than karyotyping,[25,38] but can also be associated with misclassification, particularly if maternal tissue is present. In addition, ploidy analysis cannot distinguish between a diploid molar pregnancy and hydropic abortion.[39] The most accurate is probably a multidisciplinary approach using hCG and ultrasound features in order to screen out those cases that require histology, follow up and referral. As most women in Europe and North America now have access to an ultrasound examination in early pregnancy, women presenting with ultrasound features suggesting a hydatidiform mole should be fully investigated including cytogenetic or ploidy analysis and detailed histopathology. Women could be further selected for this investigation before a uterine evacuation on the basis of their serum hCG level but this screening strategy needs to be tested prospectively.

Rare causes of true PHM

Villous hydatidiform transformation can be found in association with tetraploidy and other chromosomal abnormalities.[32] As the vast majority of tetraploidies miscarry spontaneously during the first weeks of pregnancy, tetraploidies resulting from a double or triple paternal contribution and presenting with a partial 'molar' placenta have been rarely described in ongoing pregnancies. Confined placental diploid or triploid mosaicism may appear as triploid partial mole on scan but in these cases, the fetus is anatomically normal and has a diploid karyotype.[32] Ultrasound and pathological examination may in rare cases be complicated by the fact that the molar placental tissue comes from a resorbed twin. In these cases, the mother remains at risk for the complications of triploid PHM and in particular she may subsequently develop early PIH. In most of these cases, the MShCG is high[34] and the mother is at risk of pGTD.

Pseudo-PHM

In missed miscarriage, independently of the presence of a chromosomal abnormality, the progressive disappearance of the villous vasculature after embryonic death (before 7–8 weeks' menstrual age) leads to villous hydrops, which does not however herald a true PHM.[17] Focal villous hydropic changes may also be found in pregnancies presenting with trisomy or monosomy and are probably related to insufficient development of the villous vasculature in some placental areas as part of a larger vascular maldevelopment involving the fetal circulation or to villous degeneration in cases of placental retention following embryonic/fetal demise. Hydrops of the stem villi with placentomegaly but a normal trophoblast have also been observed in cases of Beckwith–Wiedemann syndrome and with a phenotypically normal fetus. This anomaly appears to be a limited malformation of the extraembryonic mesoderm involving the mesenchyme and the vessels of the stem villi of several cotyledons and it has, therefore, been referred to as mesenchymal dysplasia. Beside a partial mole appearance and increased thickness, the placenta show no vascular abnormalities until mid-gestation. Overall, the risk of pGTD developing from a histologically confirmed nonmolar hydropic miscarriage is considered to be less than 1 in 50 000.[40]

Invasive hydatidiform mole

An invasive mole is defined as the penetration of molar villi from a CHM or PHM into the myometrium or the uterine vasculature.[32] Rarely, the molar tissue can penetrate the whole thickness of the myometrium (percreta) leading to uterine perforation and/or local pelvic extension. In contrast to choriocarcinoma, an invasive mole contains villus structures with a variable degree of trophoblastic proliferation and produces a lower level of hCG. An invasive mole usually becomes clinically apparent after the evacuation of a molar pregnancy, the woman usually presenting with heavy vaginal bleeding. The tumour appears sonographically as focal areas of increased echogenicity within the myometrium. These nodules usually appear several weeks after evacuation of a mole but may occur concurrently with a mole. The sonographic features of these nodules are similar to the lesions found in cases of placental-site trophoblastic tumours.[32] In both GTDs, the lesions are usually heterogeneous and often contain fluid-filled cavities. An early diagnosis allowing immediate treatment may, in some cases, prevent uterine perforation and the need to perform a hysterectomy.

Intrauterine pGTD

Nodules of residual GTD are surrounded by newly formed vessels with frequent arteriovenous anastomosis which produce a characteristic ultrasound pattern.[32] The most frequent feature is hypoechoic areas (blood lacunae) surrounded by irregular echogenic areas (trophoblastic nodules) and numerous intramyometrial signals (vascular shunts). In these cases, Doppler investigations of the uterine vasculature and of small intratumoral vessels have consistently shown a low impedance to flow and high peak systolic velocities. Small nodules may not be detected by Doppler imaging and hysteroscopy[41] and possibly sonohysterography may be of clinical use in women with hCG levels suggestive of persistent GTD but a negative ultrasound examination.

CONCLUSIONS

A proportion of molar pregnancies will be associated with persistent trophoblastic disease and therefore serum hCG follow up in these women is essential. The length of follow up varies depending on the rate of resolution of serum hCG levels – thus ongoing review in tertiary referral GTD units is the cornerstone of management. Histological and not ultrasound diagnosis is the gold standard prior to labelling a woman with a molar pregnancy and all its sequelae.

PRACTICAL POINTS

1. Both complete and partial molar pregnancies are associated with persistent trophoblastic disease (10–20% and 0.1–11%, respectively) and therefore should be followed up with serum hCG levels.
2. Ultrasound diagnosis of complete mole can be made in around 80% of the cases.
3. Ultrasound diagnosis of partial mole is less accurate and around 70% of those cases will be missed.
4. Although ultrasound can be helpful in the diagnosis of molar pregnancies, histological confirmation is mandatory.
5. Classically, women with singleton complete molar pregnancies present with vaginal bleeding, uterine enlargement greater than expected for gestational age and an abnormally high level of serum hCG.
6. Medical complications of molar pregnancy include pregnancy-induced hypertension, hyperthyroidism, hyperemesis gravidarum, anaemia and the development of ovarian theca lutein cyst.
7. Early diagnosis of invasive hydatidiform mole can prevent uterine perforation and the need to perform a hysterectomy.

REFERENCES

1. Kim S. Epidemiology. In: Hancock BW, Newlands ES, Berkowitz RS (eds). Gestational Trophoblastic Disease. London: Chapman & Hall, 1997: 27–42
2. Berkowitz RS, Goldstein DP. Chorionic tumors. N Engl J Med 1996; 335:1740–8.
3. Jeffers MD, O'Dwyer P, Curran B, et al. Partial hydatidiform mole: A common but underdiagnosed condition. Int J Gynecol Pathol 1993; 12:315–23.
4. Palmer JR. Advances in the epidemiology of gestational trophoblastic tumors. J Reprod Med 1994; 39:155–162.
5. Fukunaga M. Early partial hydatidiform mole: prevalence, histopathology, DNA ploidy and persistence rate. Virchows Arch 2000; 437:180–4.
6. Seckl MJ, Fisher RA, Salerno G, et al. Choriocarcinoma and partial hydatidiform moles. Lancet 2000; 1 36–9.
7. Jauniaux E, Nicolaides KH. Early ultrasound diagnosis and follow-up of molar pregnancies. Ultrasound Obstet Gynecol 1997; 9:17–21.

8. Lindholm H, Flam F. The diagnosis of molar pregnancy by sonography and gross morphology. Acta Obstet Gynecol Scand 1999; 78:6–9.

9. Lazarus E, Hulka CA, Siewert B, et al. Sonographic appearance of early complete molar pregnancies. J Ultrasound Med 1999; 18:589–93.

10. Benson CB, Genest DR, Bernstein MR, et al. Sonographic appearance of first trimester complete hydatidiform moles. Ultrasound Obstet Gynecol 2000; 16:188–91.

11. Jauniaux E. Diagnosis and management of trophoblastic and non-trophoblastic tumours. In: Kingdom J, Jauniaux E, O'Brien S (eds). The Placenta: Basic Science and Clinical Practice. London: RCOG Press; 2000: 221–37.

12. Johns J, Greenwold N, Buckley S, et al. Ultrasound in the screening and diagnosis of molar pregnancies in miscarriages. Ultrasound Obstet Gynecol 2005; 25(5):493–7.

13. Szulman AE, Surti U. The syndromes of hydatidiform mole. I. Cytogenetic and morphologic correlations. Am J Obstet Gynecol 1978; 131:665–71.

14. Szulman AE, Surti U. The syndromes of hydatidiform mole. II. Morphologic evolution of complete and partial mole. Am J Obstet Gynecol 1978; 132:20–7.

15. Szulman AE, Philippe E, Boue JG, et al. Human triploidy: Association with partial hydatidiform moles and non-molar conceptuses. Hum Pathol 1981; 12:1016–21.

16. Paradinas FJ. The diagnosis and prognosis of molar pregnancy: The experience of the National Referral Centre in London. Int J Gynaecol Obstet 1998; 60:S57–S64.

17. Jauniaux E. Partial moles: from postnatal to prenatal diagnosis. Placenta 1999; 20:379–88.

18. Kajii T, Ohama K. Androgenetic origin of hydatidiform mole. Nature 1977; 268:633–4.

19. Jauniaux E, Kadri R, Hustin J. Partial mole and triploidy: screening patients with first trimester spontaneous abortion. Obstet Gynecol 1996; 88:616–19.

20. Jauniaux E, Hustin J. Histological examination of first trimester spontaneous abortions: The impact of materno-embryonic interface features. Histopathology 1992; 21:409–14.

21. Jacobs PA, Szulman AE, Funkhouser J, et al. Human triploidy: relationship between parental origin of the additional haploid complement and development of partial hydatidiform mole. Ann Hum Genet 1982; 46:223–31.

22. McFadden DE, Kwong LC, Yam IYL, et al. Parental origin of triploidy in human fetuses: evidence from genomic imprinting. Hum Genet 1993; 92:465–9.

23. Szulman AE, Surti U. The clinicopathologic profile of the partial hydatidiform mole. Obstet Gynecol 1982; 59:597–602.

24. Zaragoza MV, Surti U, Redline RW, et al. Parental origin and phenotype of triploidy in spontaneous abortions: Predominance of diandry and association with partial hydatidiform mole. Am J Hum Genet 2000; 66:1807–20.

25. Fukunaga M. Early partial hydatidiform moles: Prevalence, histopathology, DNA ploidy, and persistence rate. Virchows Arch 2000; 437:180–4.

26. Jauniaux E, Gulbis B, Hyett J, et al. Biochemical analyses of mesenchymal fluid in early pregnancy. Am J Obstet Gynecol 1998; 178:765–9.

27. Heath V, Chadwick V, Cook I, et al. Should tissue from pregnancy termination and uterine evacuation routinely be examined histologically? Br J Obstet Gynecol 2000; 107:727–30.

28. Seckl MJ, Gillmore R, Foskett M, et al. Routine terminations of pregnancy – should we screen for gestational trophoblastic neoplasia? Lancet 2004; 364:705–7.

29. Jauniaux E, Burton GJ. Pathophysiology of histological changes in early pregnancy loss. Placenta 2005; 26:114–23.

30. Bagshawe KD, Lawler SD, Paradinas FJ, et al. Gestational trophoblastic tumours following initial diagnosis of partial hydatidiform mole. Lancet 1990; 335:1074–6.

31. Chen RJ, Huang SC, Chow SN, et al. Persistent gestational trophoblastic tumour with partial hydatidiform mole as the antecedent pregnancy. Br J Obstet Gynaecol 1994; 101:330–4.

32. Jauniaux E. Ultrasond diagnosis and follow-up of gestational trophoblastic disease. Ultrasound Obstet Gynecol 1998; 11:367–77.

33. Jauniaux E, Brown R, Snijders RJM, Noble P, Nicolaides K. Early prenatal diagnosis of triploidy. Am J Obstet Gynecol 1997; 176:550–4.

34. Jauniaux E, Bersinger NA, Gulbis B, Meuris S. The contribution of maternal serum markers in the early prenatal diagnosis of molar pregnancies. Hum Reprod 1999; 14;842.

35. Jauniaux E, Gavriil P, Khun P, et al., Fetal heart rate and umbilicoplacental Doppler flow velocity waveforms in early pregnancies with a chromosomal abnormality and/or increased nuchal translucency thickness. Hum Reprod 1996; 11:435–9.

36. Naumoff P, Szulman AE, Weinstein B, et al. Ultrasonography of partial hydatidiform mole. Radiology 1981; 140:467–70.

37. Fine C, Bundy AL, Berkowitz RS, et al. Sonographic diagnosis of partial hydatidiform mole. Obstet Gynecol 1989; 73:414–18.

38. Genest DR. Partial hydatidiform mole: clinicopathological features, differential diagnosis, ploidy, molecular studies and gold standards for diagnosis. Int J Gynecol Pathol 2001; 20:315–22.

39. Bell KA, Van Deerlin V, Addya K, et al. Molecular genetic testing from paraffin embedded tissue distinguishes nonmolar hydropic abortion from hydatidiform mole. Mol Diagn 1999; 4:11–19.

40. Sebire NJ, Foskett M, Fisher RA, et al. Persistent gestational trophoblastic disease is rarely, if ever, derived from non-molar first-trimester miscarriage. Med Hypotheses. 2005; 64:689–93.

41. Lindholm H, Radestad A, Flam F. Hysteroscopy provides proof of trophoblastic tumors in three cases with negative color Doppler images. Ultrasound Obstet Gynecol 1997; 9:59–61.

15

The management of ovarian cysts in early pregnancy

George Condous

Introduction • Expectant management • Risk of torsion • Case report 1 • Case report 2 • Conclusion • Practical points

INTRODUCTION

Prevalence

The prevalence of adnexal pathology in the first trimester has been reported as varying from 0.2% to 5.4%.[1-4] In a recent cross-sectional study, the prevalence of ovarian cysts at various stages of pregnancy was assessed, i.e. in the first, second and third trimesters. Only 1.2% (79/6636) of the total number of women in this study had an ovarian cyst with a maximum diameter of greater than 30 mm.[3] This figure was significantly lower than in a more recent longitudinal study in which the prevalence of ovarian cysts of ≥25 mm in the first trimester was 5.4% (161/3000).[4] This difference in prevalence most likely reflects the different cut-off values used as inclusion criteria in these studies and the timing of the scans. In the paper by Condous et al. transvaginal scans (TVS) were performed in the first trimester, when one would expect the presence of more physiological ovarian cysts, such as functional corpora lutea. After 16 weeks' gestation the prevalence of ovarian cysts is reported to be between 0.5% and 3.0%.[2,3] In our longitudinal study, the prevalence of ovarian cysts beyond 16 weeks' gestation was 0.9%, which is in keeping with these previous reports. In short, as the pregnancy advances, the prevalence of ovarian cysts falls.

Natural history of ovarian cysts diagnosed in early pregnancy

In the largest prospective observational longitudinal study to date, 3000 women underwent TVS in the first trimester. This study differed from previous cross sectional studies in that the prevalence of ovarian pathology was established in an early pregnancy population and then the natural history of the ovarian cysts in these women was observed. Although 6.1% of women were found to have an ovarian cyst of ≥25 mm, complete follow-up data were available on 5.4%.[4] The mean gestational age at the time of diagnosis was 53 days (7 weeks and 4 days). These women were scanned every 4–6 weeks throughout the pregnancy (transabdominal scans were performed after 14 weeks' gestation) until resolution of the ovarian cyst occurred, intervention was required or the pregnancy concluded. Intervention was required if the ovarian cyst was causing symptoms of pain as a result of presumed subacute or acute torsion; or if the ovarian cyst was thought to be suspicious in nature according to the ultrasonographic appearance. The results showed that 119/166 (71.7%) of the ovarian cysts resolved spontaneously – these were classified as cystic or haemorrhagic corpus lutea based upon the greyscale ultrasound appearance.[4] If we excluded the complex ovarian cysts, as many as 86.9% of simple or

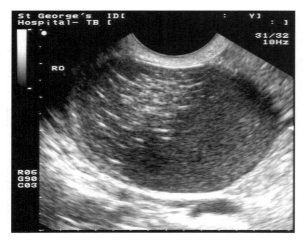

Figure 15.1 Benign teratoma of the ovary.

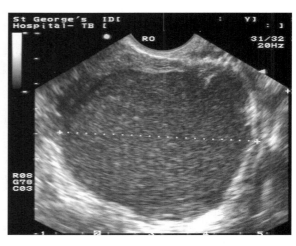

Figure 15.2 Endometrioma.

haemorrhagic ovarian cysts resolved sponta-neously.[4] Forty out of 166 (24.1%) persisted 6 weeks after the pregnancy concluded. Interestingly, if an ovarian cyst was present at 20 weeks' gestation, 78.6% of these persisted at the 6-week postnatal scan and all were patho-logical.[4] Seven out of 166 (4.2%) required treat-ment and only four of these required acute intervention.[4]

As only 0.13% (1.3/1000) of women with an ovarian cyst in this study required acute inter-vention (during the course of the pregnancy), we concluded that examining the ovaries at the time of a first-trimester scan is of limited value.[4] Those women requiring intervention will present with abdominal pain in any event, whilst prior knowledge of the presence of an ovarian cyst may only increase anxiety even though the risk of complication is very low. If a non-malignant-looking ovarian cyst is noted at the time of a first-trimester ultrasound scan, we recommend that these women should be offered a follow-up scan 6 weeks after the pregnancy has concluded.

Classification of ovarian cysts with ultrasound scan

Data relating to the morphological characteri-zation and subjective assessment of ovarian masses have been well documented.[5–8] Ovarian masses can be accurately classified according to the ultrasound appearance and therefore appro-priate management can be made on the basis of this.[5–8] The subjective assessment of ultrasound images has been shown to be highly predictive for both malignant and benign adnexal masses.[7] In the same study, the first ultrasonographer and the most experienced investigator both obtained an accuracy of 92%. There was very good agreement between these two investiga-tors in the classification of the adnexal masses (Cohen's kappa 0.85). The less-experienced observers obtained a significantly lower accuracy, which varied between 82% and 87%. Their interobserver agreement was moderate to good (Cohen's kappa 0.52–0.76).[7] In the few cases where the nature of an ovarian cyst is in question, one must balance the risks to the pregnancy from intervention versus the risk of malignancy based on the ultrasound scan.[7]

It is well accepted that 10% of adnexal masses are extremely difficult to classify.[7] In the author's study, three women fell into this category and were thought to have borderline lesions based upon the ultrasonographic appearance, i.e. the presence of papillary projections that were non-vascular with colour Doppler. Only one of these was confirmed histologically – the others were a benign cystic

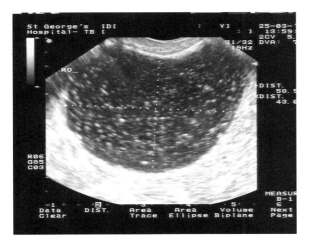

Figure 15.3 Mucinous cystadenoma of the ovary.

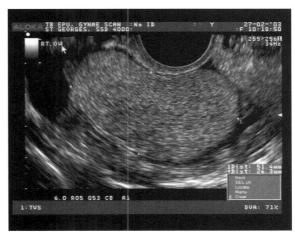

Figure 15.4 Benign teratoma of the ovary.

teratoma and a benign haemorrhagic ovarian cyst that had undergone torsion. This highlights the difficulty in classifying some ovarian masses.

Risk of ovarian malignancy in pregnancy

The incidence of ovarian malignancy in pregnancy is extremely rare – it is reported to be between 1 in 15 000 and 1 in 32 000 pregnancies.[9] Women with ovarian cysts that have ultrasound features suggestive of malignancy diagnosed in the first trimester should be referred for a gynaecological oncology opinion with a view to considering intervention after 14 weeks' gestation.

In a cross-sectional study of 2245 women, there were no cases of malignancy.[1] In another study of 55 278 women undergoing termination of pregnancy, there were only two cases of ovarian malignancy.[2] In a further cross-sectional study of 6636 women, although there were no cases of ovarian invasive malignancy, three women were noted to have stage 1a borderline tumours.[3] In the author's study of 3000 women in the first trimester, there was only one borderline tumour. Despite the fact that the borderline lesion in this study was managed surgically, there is evidence to suggest that expectant management of such

ovarian cysts is an option. In a recent study by Zanetta et al.,[3] this approach to borderline ovarian lesions was shown to be safe. Three women with ovarian cysts suggestive of borderline change were managed expectantly and after the pregnancy they underwent surgery.[3] Their staging was not compromised by such management, i.e. all three tumours were stage 1a at laparotomy and subsequent histological assessment.

EXPECTANT MANAGEMENT

Because complications of abdominal surgery are increased in pregnancy, the surgical management of ovarian cysts in pregnancy has been reconsidered.[10] Historically, pregnant women with persistent adnexal masses underwent elective removal of the masses in the second trimester.[11] This is no longer acceptable practice in asymptomatic women, as surgical intervention, either as an emergency or after 24 weeks' gestation is associated with a poorer obstetric outcome.[12] Complications include spontaneous miscarriage or preterm premature rupture of membranes (PPROM).[10] In modern management, if surgery is to be performed, laparoscopic treatment of adnexal masses in the second trimester has been shown to be safe and effective.[13–15] In selected cases, close observation

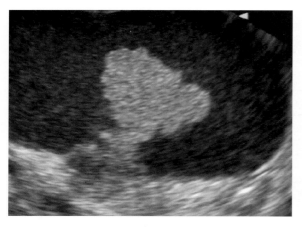

Figure 15.5 Endometrioma with solid papillary projection.

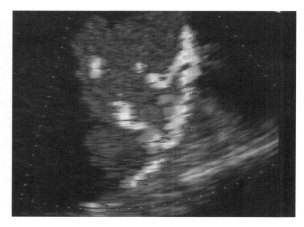

Figure 15.6 Endometrioma with vascular solid papillary projection on colour Doppler, consistent with endometrioid adenocarcinoma. (See also colour plate)

is a reasonable alternative to antenatal surgery in women with an adnexal mass during pregnancy.[16]

If the nature of an ovarian cyst diagnosed in the first trimester is not in question, expectant management of asymptomatic ovarian masses is advocated, at least until the pregnancy is beyond 14 weeks' gestation.[4,17,18] When symptomatic, simple ovarian cysts diagnosed during pregnancy can be successfully and safely treated with ultrasound guided cyst aspiration.[19] Aspiration of simple ovarian cysts during pregnancy is safe, may save surgical intervention and in some cases this will be the definitive treatment.[19] Neither anaesthesia nor analgesia are required for such intervention. Ultrasound-guided aspiration for the relief of pain generated by simple ovarian cysts in non-pregnant women can be performed either transvaginally or transabdominally depending on the cyst location.[20] After 14 weeks' gestation, the uterus is an abdominal organ and as a result the ovaries are more easily targeted transabdominally. Fine-needle aspiration is not appropriate if the cyst has any suspicious morphological features.[21]

Expectant management of women with ovarian cysts diagnosed in the first trimester should be encouraged.[4,17,18] Although there are no randomized clinical trials to determine the

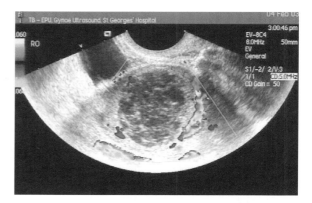

Figure 15.7 Haemorrhagic corpus luteum with 'ring of fire' demonstrated using colour Doppler. (See also colour plate)

optimal management of an adnexal mass in pregnancy, our experience suggests that expectant management is safe and without serious adverse outcome for mother and fetus. It would be ethically difficult to justify randomizing women to intervention for persistent adnexal masses. We adopted an expectant management approach to our population, and our data and others suggest that it is safe, decreases the number of unnecessary surgical interventions and is not associated with an adverse outcome.[3,4,17,18] We have developed a flow diagram for the management of asymptomatic

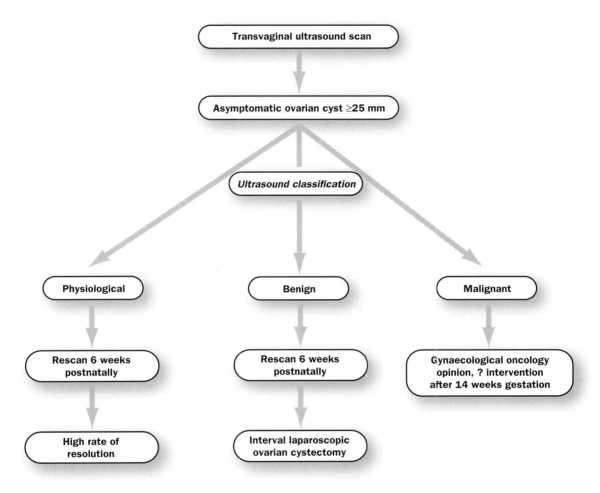

Figure 15.8 Flow diagram to illustrate a suggested management plan for women with an asymptomatic ovarian cyst in the first trimester.

ovarian cysts on the basis of our trial (Figure 15.8).

RISK OF TORSION

The rate of torsion decreases as the gestation increases. This was confirmed by the author's study in which women were recruited in the first trimester; it is not surprising that the rate of torsion (3%)[4] was higher than in the published literature (1%).[6] Ovarian torsion is difficult to diagnose at all stages of pregnancy and other causes of an acute abdomen must be excluded first. A high index of clinical suspicion

is the key to diagnosing torsion; colour Doppler does not play a decisive role. We have developed a flow diagram for the management of symptomatic ovarian cysts visualized in the first trimester (Figure 15.9).

CASE REPORT 1

A 30-year-old woman presented to the Early Pregnancy Unit in her first pregnancy at 6 weeks' gestation with vaginal spotting. She underwent a TVS and a 6 week viable intrauterine pregnancy was confirmed. She was also noted to have an incidental non-tender left

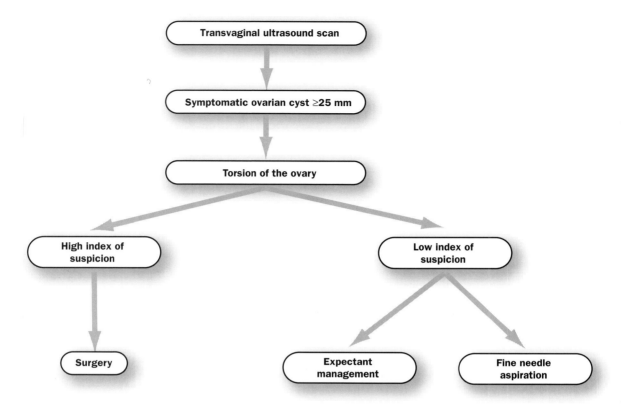

Figure 15.9 Flow diagram to illustrate a suggested management plan for women with a symptomatic ovarian cyst in the first trimester.

ovarian cyst measuring 50 × 49 × 40 mm with internal 'spider-web' echoes (see Figure 15.7); the right ovary was normal in size and appearance. A diagnosis of haemorrhagic corpus luteum was made. She was reassured about the viability of her pregnancy and the functional nature of the asymptomatic ovarian cyst. She was managed expectantly and a rescan 4 weeks later, at 10 weeks' gestation, confirmed resolution of this physiological cyst. She was reassured and she was rebooked for her nuchal scan.

CASE REPORT 2

A 35-year-old Para 2+0 woman presented at 13+3 weeks' gestation with severe lower abdominal pain. A TVS and transabdominal scan confirmed a viable 13-week fetus and she was noted to have a tender right ovarian simple cyst measuring 110 × 90 × 70 mm; the left ovary was

normal in size and appearance. A diagnosis of subacute torsion was made and she underwent transabdominal ultrasound-guided drainage of this ovarian cyst. This was done in an attempt to alleviate her symptoms and also to potentially avoid surgery. In the days following treatment, her symptoms improved dramatically. At repeat transabdominal ultrasound scan at 20 weeks' gestation, the right ovarian cyst had reformed, albeit smaller and measuring 80 × 70 × 60 mm – she was noted to be asymptomatic. A diagnosis of serous cystadenoma was made based upon the ultrasound appearance of the cyst. The persistent and benign nature of the ovarian cyst was explained to her and she was managed conservatively, with the understanding that the risk for torsion decreased as the pregnancy advanced. She was booked for a 6 week postnatal TVS. Six weeks after she had a normal vaginal delivery at term, a TVS demonstrated a persistent right ovarian simple cyst measuring $80 \times 65 \times 55$ mm. She was booked for an interval laparoscopic ovarian cystectomy because of the ongoing risk of torsion and this later confirmed a serous cystadenoma on histology and she was discharged.

CONCLUSION

Expectant management should be the accepted standard of clinical practice for the management of ovarian cysts diagnosed in the first trimester. The majority of ovarian cysts detected in the first trimester resolve spontaneously. As only 1.3/1000 women with an ovarian cyst in early pregnancy require acute intervention throughout their pregnancy, surgical intervention should be the exception rather than the rule. It is rarely indicated and should be reserved for those women with an acute abdomen or those in which there is a high index of suspicion of malignancy based on the ultrasound appearance.

If a benign ovarian cyst is noted at the time of the first-trimester ultrasound scan, these women should be reassured and offered a follow-up scan 6 weeks after the pregnancy has concluded.

PRACTICAL POINTS

1. The prevalence of adnexal pathology in the first trimester is up to 5.4%.
2. The vast majority of ovarian cysts diagnosed on ultrasound scan in the first trimester are physiological corpus lutea and resolve spontaneously.
3. Expectant management of ovarian cysts diagnosed in the first trimester should be the standard of care, if the nature of the cyst is not in question.
4. Simple ovarian cysts, when symptomatic during pregnancy, can be successfully and safely treated with ultrasound-guided cyst aspiration.
5. If surgery is to be performed, laparoscopic treatment of adnexal masses in the second trimester has been shown to be safe and effective.
6. As only 1.3/1000 women with an ovarian cyst in the first trimester require acute intervention (during the course of the pregnancy), examining the ovaries at the time of a first trimester scan is of limited value.
7. It is well accepted that 10% of adnexal masses are extremely difficult to classify using transvaginal ultrasonography.
8. The incidence of ovarian malignancy in pregnancy is extremely rare – it is reported to be between 1 in 15 000 and 1 in 32 000 pregnancies.
9. The rate of ovarian torsion decreases as the gestation increases.
10. A high index of clinical suspicion is the key to diagnosing ovarian torsion; colour Doppler does not play a decisive role.

REFERENCES

1. Czekierdowski A, Bednarek W, Rogowska W, et al. Difficulties in differential diagnosis of adnexal masses during pregnancy: the role of greyscale and color doppler sonography. Ginekology 2001; 72:1281–6.
2. Ballard CA. Ovarian tumors associated with pregnancy termination patients. Am J Obstet Gynecol 1984; 149:384–7.
3. Zanetta G, Mariani E, Lissoni A, et al. A prospective study of the role of ultrasound in the management of adnexal masses in pregnancy. Br J Obstet Gynaecol 2003; 110:578–83.
4. Condous G, Khalid A, Okaro E, et al. Should we be examining the ovaries in pregnancy? The natural history of adnexal pathology detected at first trimester ultrasonography. Ultrasound Obstet Gynecol 2004; 24:62–6.

5. Jermy K, Luise C, Bourne T. The characterization of common ovarian cysts in premenopausal women. Ultrasound Obstet Gynecol 2001; 17:140–4.

6. Bromley B, Benacerraf B. Adnexal masses during pregnancy: Accuracy of sonographic diagnosis and outcome. J Ultrasound Med 1997; 16:447–52.

7. Timmerman D, Schwarzler P, Collins WP, et al. Subjective assessment of adnexal masses with the use of ultrasonography: an analysis of interobserver variability and experience. Ultrasound Obstet Gynecol 1999; 13:11–6.

8. Timor-Tritsch LE, Lerner JP, Monteagudo A, et al. Transvaginal ultrasonographic characterization of ovarian masses by means of color flow-directed Doppler measurement and a morphological scoring system. Am J Obstet Gynecol 1993; 168:909–13.

9. Goffinet F. Ovarian cysts and pregnancy. J Gynecol Obstet Biol Reprod 2001; 30:S100–8.

10. Platek DN, Henderson CE, Goldberg GL. The management of a persistent adnexal mass in pregnancy. Am J Obstet Gynecol 1996; 173:1236–40.

11. Hess LW, Peaceman A, O'Brien WF, et al. Adnexal mass occurring with intrauterine pregnancy: report of fifty-four patients requiring laparotomy for definitive management. Am J Obstet Gynecol 1988; 158: 1029–34.

12. Agarwal N, Parul, Kriplani A, et al. Management and outcome of pregnancies complicated with adnexal masses. Arch Gynecol Obstet 2003; 267:148–52.

13. Soriano D, Yefet Y, Seidman DS, et al. Laparoscopy versus laparotomy in the management of adnexal masses during pregnancy. Fertil Steril 1999; 71:955–60.

14. Stepp KJ, Tulikangas PK, Goldberg JM, et al. Laparoscopy for adnexal masses in the second trimester of pregnancy. J Am Assoc Gynecol Laparosc 2003; 10:55–9.

15. Howard FM, Vill M. Laparoscopic adnexal surgery during pregnancy. J Am Assoc Gynecol Laparosc 1994; 2:91–3.

16. Schmeler KM, Mayo-Smith WW, Peipert JF, et al. Adnexal masses in pregnancy: surgery compared with observation. Obstet Gynecol 2005; 105:1098–103.

17. Condous G, Okaro E, Bourne T. The conservative management of early pregnancy complications: a review of the literature. Ultrasound Obstet Gynecol 2003; 22:420–30.

18. Condous G. The management of early pregnancy complications. Best Pract Res Clin Obstet Gynaecol 2004; 18:37–57.

19. Caspi B, Ben-Arie A, Appelman Z, et al. Aspiration of simple pelvic cysts during pregnancy. Gynecol Obstet Invest 2000; 49:102–5.

20. Caspi B, Zalel Y, Lurie S, et al. Ultrasound-guided aspiration for pain relief generated by simple ovarian cysts. Gynecol Obstet Invest 1993; 35:121–2.

21. Hermans RH, Fischer DC, van der Putten HW, et al. Adnexal masses in pregnancy. Onkologie 2003; 26:167–72.

16

Hyperemesis gravidarum

Maha Alkatib

Introduction • Pathophysiology • Diagnosis • Investigations • Management • Conclusions • Practical points

INTRODUCTION

Nausea and vomiting in pregnancy is a common condition affecting up to 80% of all pregnant women.[1] Hyperemesis gravidarum (HG), however, describes 0.3–1.5% of pregnancies where the severity and persistence of the vomiting results in weight loss and ketosis as a result of dehydration and nutritional deficiency.[2] Women commonly, but not exclusively, present in the first trimester after 6–8 weeks' gestation resulting in the third-leading cause for hospital admissions during pregnancy.[3] If not managed aggressively, life-threatening conditions such as Wernicke's encephalopathy, central pontine myelinosis,[4] rhabdomyolysis, peripheral neuropathy (from electrolyte and vitamin deficiencies), pneumomediastinum, Mallory–Weiss tears and oesophageal rupture (from pressures on oesophagus),[5] pulmonary embolism and deep vein thrombosis (from immobility and haemoconcentration) have been reported, ultimately resulting in maternal deaths.[6] The main impact on the fetus if electrolyte imbalances have occurred in a HG pregnancy is that of low birthweight.[7] Fetal death occurs in approximately 40% of women who develop Wernicke's encephalopathy.[4]

Table 16.1. Possible pathophysiological processes involved in hyperemesis gravidarum

Possible aetiology	Source	Pathophysiology
hCG	Placenta Corpus luteum	Distension of upper GI tract Crossover with thyroid stimulating hormone (TSH) contributing to gestational thyrotoxicosis[10]
Oestrogen/progesterone	Placenta	Decreased gut motility Elevated liver enzymes Decreased lower oesophageal sphincter pressure Elevated levels of sex steroids in hepatic portal system[11]
Helicobacter pylori	Gastrointestinal tract	Subclinical *H. pylori* activated by altered immunity in pregnancy and increased steroid levels in circulation[12]
Psychological		Suggested due to difference in incidences of HG in different populations/cultures and improvement when taken away from environmental influences[13]

PATHOPHYSIOLOGY

This is still poorly understood, the most common theory suggests a direct link with the serum human chorionic gonadotrophin (hCG) levels which peak at 6–12 weeks' gestation and is higher in multiple pregnancies and molar pregnancies where hyperemesis is more prevalent.[8] Interestingly more female infants are born to women with HG earlier on in pregnancy.[9] Table 16.1 highlights all the current theories proposed to be involved in the pathogenesis of HG.

DIAGNOSIS

HG is a diagnosis of exclusion and usually does not present with significant abdominal pain. A history of HG in previous pregnancies increases the likelihood of recurrence. Other causes of vomiting in pregnancy should be ruled out first.

Infection

Urinary tract infection is a common explanation for excessive vomiting in pregnancy. Others such as hepatitis, meningitis or gastroenteritis should also be considered although they may present with associated abdominal pain/neurological symptoms.

Gastrointestinal

Appendicitis, cholecystitis, pancreatitis, fatty liver, peptic ulceration and small bowel obstruction can present with vomiting – abdominal pain is also a key finding in such cases.

Metabolic

Biochemical thyrotoxicosis is seen in women with HG (~60%) and more commonly in women from the Asian sub-continent.[14,15] The aetiology is uncertain and the finding is self-limiting with improvement in serum levels once the vomiting has settled. Symptoms predating the pregnancy should be looked for to distinguish this from pre-existing Grave's disease.

Addison's disease, diabetic ketoacidosis and hyperparathyroidism, albeit rare, can present with vomiting and should be considered when performing investigations.

Drugs

Various medications may induce vomiting, typically antibiotics and iron supplements taken regularly by pregnant women.

INVESTIGATIONS

Biochemical investigations should include serum urea and electrolytes, liver function tests, thyroid function tests and serum hCG levels. In HG hyponatraemia, hypokalaemia and low serum urea are seen. A metabolic hypochloraemic alkalosis is also encountered. Approximately 15–25% of women will have abnormal liver function tests, including elevated transaminases and a mildly raised bilirubin insufficient to cause jaundice (resolves once hyperemesis is treated).[16] A biochemical thyrotoxicosis showing elevated thyroxine and suppressed TSH levels as mentioned before is seen in most HG cases. Reference ranges for pregnant women should be used as baseline levels do change in every trimester, and appear abnormal compared to non-pregnant ranges.

Haematological investigations should concentrate specifically at the haematocrit level which will be raised in HG.

Urinalysis usually reveals ketonuria and will help exclude a urinary tract infection.

Ultrasound of the pregnancy, whether transvaginal or transabdominal, is performed to determine gestation, number of fetuses and to exclude a molar pregnancy. However, in a recent study, pregnancies complicated by HG had a similar risk of twin pregnancy, and a lower risk of early pregnancy failure compared to controls.[17] In the absence of vaginal bleeding, there was no increase in gestational trophoblastic disease in women with HG. Kirk et al concluded that an ultrasound scan is not clinically necessary in women presenting with HG, other than for maternal reassurance.[17]

MANAGEMENT

Admission is usually necessary if there is ketosis and there is an inability to rehydrate orally due to intractable vomiting. Baseline observations including pulse rate, postural blood pressure and weight should be recorded. Given the generally fatigued state women are admitted in, immobility is likely and bed rest encouraged, hence thromboprophylaxis in the form of thromboembolic stockings or low-molecular-weight heparin should be commenced.

Rehydration

Aggressive rehydration is the mainstay of treatment in HG with women noticing an improvement in wellbeing despite any other interventions. Sodium-containing crystalloid solutions, i.e. normal saline or Hartmann's solution have adequate amounts of sodium to replenish any existing hyponatraemia. Double-strength saline should be avoided due to the risk of central pontine myelinosis developing from rapid correction of hyponatraemia. Dextrose-containing solutions are to be avoided at all times due to the risk of the dextrose precipitating Wernicke's encephalopathy. Potassium supplementation in the intravenous fluids should be added and titrated according to the deficiency seen on serum measurements.

The rate of infusion of fluids is dependent upon the degree of electrolyte imbalance, the degree of ketosis and the oral intake and output of fluid. Usually on admission this would involve rapid infusion rates of 1 litre per 2–4-hourly frequencies due to being in a negative fluid balance state. Changes in weight help to determine the adequacy of rehydration and modification of the regime if warranted.

Thromboprophylaxis

Given the potential haemoconcentrating effect of dehydration and immobility of women affected by HG, thromboprophylaxis is recommended. This should be, as a minimum, in the form of thromboembolic stockings, and if a raised haematocrit is encountered, include prophylactic doses of low-molecular-weight heparin.

Vitamin supplementation

Thiamine deficiency may be encountered in HG which, if left untreated, can lead to Wernicke's encephalopathy. Supplementation should be prescribed on admission either orally or intravenously.

Folic acid supplementation should not be neglected in women with HG as they are commonly in their first trimester at presentation. Higher oral doses should be considered to ensure adequate absorption to prevent neural tube defects in the fetus.

Antiemetic therapy

If symptoms do not resolve with fluid and vitamin replacement alone, then antiemetic therapy can be added. This can be from a selection of pharmacological groups including antihistamines, phenothiazines, dopamine antagonists and serotonin (5HT3) antagonists. None of these have been found to have any teratogenic effects on the fetus and can be offered on a regular basis although ondansetron should be used with caution and reserved for refractory cases due to its unknown effects in the first trimester.[18] Drowsiness, oculogyric crises and extrapyramidal effects can be precipitated by phenothiazines, with metoclopramide also able to cause oculogyric crises.

Ranitidine

Histamine 2-receptor antagonists such as ranitidine are given in cases where reflux oesophagitis is suspected and can provide symptom relief. Omeprazole, a proton pump inhibitor, has also been used as an alternative and is safe in pregnancy.

Corticosteroid therapy

In cases where HG is refractory to the above treatment modalities, corticosteroid therapy has been suggested with improvement seen in severe cases.[19] The treatment course may be over a long period and the susceptibility to other infections and gestational diabetes during pregnancy needs to be made clear.

Total parenteral feeding (TPN)

If all pharmacological approaches fail then there is a pressing need to provide nutrition.

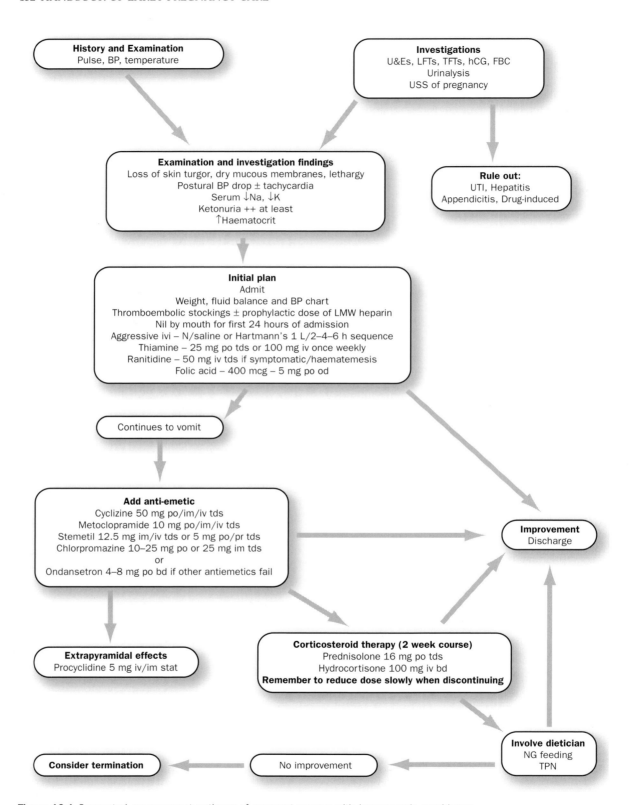

History and Examination
Pulse, BP, temperature

Investigations
U&Es, LFTs, TFTs, hCG, FBC
Urinalysis
USS of pregnancy

Examination and investigation findings
Loss of skin turgor, dry mucous membranes, lethargy
Postural BP drop ± tachycardia
Serum ↓Na, ↓K
Ketonuria ++ at least
↑Haematocrit

Rule out:
UTI, Hepatitis
Appendicitis, Drug-induced

Initial plan
Admit
Weight, fluid balance and BP chart
Thromboembolic stockings ± prophylactic dose of LMW heparin
Nil by mouth for first 24 hours of admission
Aggressive ivi – N/saline or Hartmann's 1 L/2–4–6 h sequence
Thiamine – 25 mg po tds or 100 mg iv once weekly
Ranitidine – 50 mg iv tds if symptomatic/haematemesis
Folic acid – 400 mcg – 5 mg po od

Continues to vomit

Add anti-emetic
Cyclizine 50 mg po/im/iv tds
Metoclopramide 10 mg po/im/iv tds
Stemetil 12.5 mg im/iv tds or 5 mg po/pr tds
Chlorpromazine 10–25 mg po or 25 mg im tds
or
Ondansetron 4–8 mg po bd if other antiemetics fail

Improvement
Discharge

Extrapyramidal effects
Procyclidine 5 mg iv/im stat

Corticosteroid therapy (2 week course)
Prednisolone 16 mg po tds
Hydrocortisone 100 mg iv bd
Remember to reduce dose slowly when discontinuing

Involve dietician
NG feeding
TPN

Consider termination

No improvement

Figure 16.1 Suggested management pathway of pregnant women with hyperemesis gravidarum

Nasogastric feeding is an option to consider but is usually poorly tolerated due to continuing nausea and vomiting, tube displacement and risk of aspiration. TPN is found to have a supportive effect and can be therapeutic in some cases of severe HG. Given that the route of administration requires a long line into a large vein over a long period of time, susceptibility to line infections, thrombophlebitis and bacterial endocarditis are recognized complications.[20]

Psychological support

During this period of HG there may well be recurrent admissions involving separation from family. There is also the sense of disappointment felt in some women who had had higher expectations of their pregnancy and sought an idealistic experience throughout, and yet ultimately rejection of their fetus occurred. Support from a women's counsellor in the hospital may offer help in motivating such women if these feelings have been identified by those caring for her.

Alternative therapies

Oral ginger regimens, acupuncture, diazepam and vitamin B6 therapy have all been suggested as effective alternative regimes.[21–23] Although these may offer significant improvement in nausea and vomiting in pregnancy, they have yet to be proved as an effective treatment method for HG.

Termination of pregnancy

If all modalities fail and there is a significant risk to maternal wellbeing, or if the woman is no longer able to proceed with the pregnancy in their current state, then a termination of pregnancy may be the only available option.

Figure 16.1 shows a suggested management pathway in the care of women with HG.

CONCLUSIONS

Hyperemesis gravidarum is a diagnosis of exclusion and if treated appropriately, serious sequelae can be avoided. The mainstay of treatment for women with hyperemesis gravidarum is rehydration and controlling of symptoms. Most women will have a singleton pregnancy, however an ultrasound scan should be arranged in order to exclude conditions such as multiple pregnancy or molar pregnancy.

PRACTICAL POINTS

1. Hyperemesis gravidarum complicates a small proportion of all pregnancies but has life-threatening implications if not treated early and aggressively.
2. Hyperemesis gravidarum is a diagnosis of exclusion.
3. Intravenous fluid therapy, vitamin supplementation and antiemetic therapy is the mainstay of treatment with corticosteroid therapy and TPN reserved for more resistant cases.
4. Thromboprophylaxis should always be remembered in cases where prolonged hospital admission and immobility are likely.
5. Folate supplementation is important in hyperemesis gravidarum as nutrition deficiency is a major problem.

REFERENCES

1. Gadsby R, Barnie-Adshead AM, Jagger C. A prospective study of nausea and vomiting during pregnancy. Br J Gen Pract 1993; 43:245–8.
2. Tsang IS, Katz VL, Wells SD. Maternal and fetal outcomes in hyperemesis gravidarum. Int J Gynaecol Obstet 1996; 55:231–5.
3. Bennett TA, Kotelchuck M, Cox CE. Pregnancy-associated hospitalisations in the United States in 1991 and 1992: a comprehensive review of maternal morbidity. Am J Obstet Gynecol 1998; 178:346–54.

4. Bergin PS, Harvey P. Wernicke's encephalopathy and central pontine myelinolysis with hyperemesis gravidarum. BMJ 1992; 305:517–8.

5. Liang SG, Sadovnick AD, Remick RA. Pneumomediastinum following oesophageal rupture associated with hyperemesis gravidarum. J Obstet Gynaecol Res 2002; 28:172–5.

6. Lewis G, Drife J. Why mothers die. Report on Confidential Enquiries into Maternal Deaths in the United Kingdom 1994–1996. London: The Stationery Office, 1998.

7. Kallen B. Hyperemesis during pregnancy and delivery outcome: a registry study. Eur J Obstet Gynecol Reprod Biol 1987; 26:291–302.

8. Goodwin TM, Hersham JM, Cole L. Increased concentration of the free beta-subunit of human chorionic gonadotropin in hyperemesis gravidarum. Acta Obstet Gynecol Scand 1994; 73:770–2.

9. Basso O, Olsen J. Sex ratio and twinning in women with hyperemesis or pre-eclampsia. Epidemiology 2001; 12:747–9.

10. Panesar NS, Li CY, Rogers MS. Are thyroid hormones or hCG responsible for hyperemesis gravidarum? A matched paired study in pregnant Chinese women. Acta Obstet Gynecol Scand 2001; 80:519–24.

11. Jarnfelt-Samsioe A, Bremme K, Eneroth P. Steroid hormones in emetic and non-emetic pregnancy. Eur J Obstet Gynecol Reprod Biol 1986; 21:87–99.

12. Bagis T, Gumurdulu Y, Kayaselcuk F. Endoscopy in hyperemesis gravidarum and *Helicobacter pylori* infection. Int J Gynaecol Obstet 2002; 79:105–9.

13. Swallow BL, Lindow SW, Masson EA. Psychological health in early pregnancy: relationship with nausea and vomiting. J Obstet Gynaecol 2004; 24:28–32.

14. Price A, Davies R, Heller SR. Asian women are at increased risk of gestational thyrotoxicosis. J Clin Endocrinol Metab 1996; 81:1160–3.

15. Goodwin TM, Montero M, Mestman JH. Transient hyperthyroidism and hyperemesis gravidarum: clinical aspects. Am J Obstet Gynecol 1992; 167:648–52.

16. Morali GA, Braverman DZ. Abnormal liver enzymes and ketonuria in hyperemesis gravidarum. A retrospective view of 80 patients. J Clin Gastroeneterol 1990; 12:303–5.

17. Kirk E, Papageorghiou AT, Condous G, Bottomley C, Bourne T. Hyperemesis gravidarum: is an ultrasound scan necessary? Hum Reprod 2006; in press.

18. Tincello DG, Johnstone MJ. Treatment of hyperemesis gravidarum with the 5-HT3 antagonist ondansetron. Postgrad Med J 1996; 72:688–9.

19. Nelson-Piercy C, Fayers P, de Sweit M. Randomised, double-blind, placebo-controlled trial of corticosteroids for the treatment of hyperemesis gravidarum. BJOG 2001; 108:9–15.

20. Levine MG, Esser D. TPN for the treatment of severe hyperemesis gravidarum: maternal nutritional effects and fetal outcome. Obstet Gynecol 1988; 72:102–7.

21. Vutayavanich T, Kraisarin T, Ruangsri R. Ginger for nausea and vomiting in pregnancy: randomised double-masked, placebo-controlled trial. Obstet Gynecol 2001; 97:577–82.

22. Ditto A, Morgante G, la Marca A. Evaluation of treatment of hyperemesis gravidarum using parenteral fluid with or without diazepam. A randomised study. Gynecol Obstet Invest 1999; 48:232–6.

23. Jewell D, Young G. Interventions for nausea and vomiting in early pregnancy. Cochrane Database Syst Rev 2000; 2:CD000145.

Index